How to Live a Longer, Healthier Life

WHAT REALLY MATTERS

Published by REDSG Publishing Columbia, South Carolina
Cover design and interior layout by Diana Wade Designs

ISBN 979-8-9960162-0-4

The information contained in this book is intended for general informational purposes only and should not be construed as medical advice from the author. This book is not intended to serve as a replacement for personal medical advice provided by your treating physician. All matters pertaining to your physical health should be supervised by your own health care providers. These p rofessionals can provide you with the medical care that is most appropriate for your individual needs and your particular set of clinical and personal circumstances. You should never make treatment decisions on your own without consulting your physician. Any treatment decisions should be made after joint discussions between you, your family, and your treatment team. This book is r ecommended a s a r esource for these joint discussions. However, the information, research, and suggestions for management may not be appropriate for all patients. Therefore, a health care professional should be consulted regarding your specific situation, and the author is not liable for any medical decisions made based on the contents of this book. Any use of the information contained in this book is at the reader's discretion, and the author specifically disclaims any and all liability arising directly or indirectly from the use or application of any information contained in this book, including but not limited to any actual, special, incidental, consequential, or any other form of damages and/or liability.

How to Live a Longer, Healthier Life

WHAT REALLY MATTERS

STEVEN ROSANSKY

Preface

"Do not regret growing older.
It is a privilege denied to many." - Unknown

Aging is a privilege. It is also, far more than most people realize, within our control. That is the central message of this book — and it is a message that runs against the grain of what most people believe.

There are a great many false beliefs about aging and about what it takes to live a longer, healthier life. This book is an attempt to replace those beliefs with the best available evidence — and to show that the choices within your reach matter far more than the hand you were dealt.

The picture of aging as a steady, inevitable decline simply does not reflect the science. A global survey of more than 40,000 people across 166 countries found that 80 percent of the general public believed dementia is a normal part of aging. It is not. The vast majority of older people do not develop cognitive impairment and do not need assistance to function. A separate study that followed more than 11,000 adults aged

65 and older for up to 12 years found that 45 percent showed measurable improvement in cognitive function, physical function, or both. My hope is that after reading this book, you will be one of those people - someone who actually improves in physical and cognitive function as the years go by.

Two of the most powerful forces in health and longevity are also among the least appreciated. The first is social connectedness (see Chapter 18). The evidence that meaningful relationships protect against disease, cognitive decline, and early death is as strong as the evidence for many of the medications we prescribe — and it comes without side effects. The second is the mind-body connection. Research consistently shows that how you think about aging shapes how you age: people who hold positive expectations about growing older live measurably longer, recover faster from illness, and engage more fully in the habits that protect their health. When you hold an accurate, evidence-based view of what is possible, the choices in this book become not a burden but an opportunity. This book brings together the best available evidence on the lifestyle changes and medical treatments that genuinely extend life and protect health — translated into plain language, stripped of jargon, and organized for practical use. It covers every major body system, addressing both how to prevent disease and how to manage it when it arrives. My goals are straightforward. I want you to feel less afraid of aging and more confident in your ability to shape it. I want to give you the tools to ask better questions, make more informed decisions, and push back on treatments that are expensive, unproven, or unnecessarily risky. Most of all, I want to help you not only add years to your life, but — more importantly — add years to your health span: your healthy, functional years.

Introduction

EVERY WEEK, A NEW superfood. Every month, a new supplement. Every year, a new "revolutionary" therapy that promises to reverse aging, melt fat, or prevent cancer—usually backed by a small study, a celebrity endorsement, or nothing at all. If you have spent any time trying to sort real health information from noise, you know how exhausting it is. This book is designed to end that exhaustion. My goal is not to overwhelm you with information—it is to give you the specific, reliable facts that actually can make a difference in how long and how well you live.

I have spent four decades as a physician watching this problem from the inside. As a practitioner of internal medicine and nephrology, I have cared for patients whose heart attacks, strokes, kidney failure, and amputations might have been prevented with the lifestyle choices and medical interventions that I share in this book. But I have also watched medicine harm the very patients it means to help.

In nephrology, I watched colleagues start patients on dialysis far earlier than necessary — a painful, life-altering treatment — on the assumption that an earlier start was better. My own research challenged that assumption. In a landmark study, we demonstrated that patients who began dialysis at lower levels of remaining kidney function often lived longer than those who started sooner. Dialysis was not the only problem. The business of medicine routinely overuses invasive procedures and promotes expensive interventions that lack solid evidence to support them.

To bring the truth about early dialysis initiation directly to patients, I wrote my first book, Learn the Facts About Kidney Disease. It launched at the height of the COVID-19 pandemic, and the cancellations that followed — book tours, conferences, in-person events — made it difficult to reach the audience I had written it for.

My luck changed when I connected with James Fabin, a kidney patient and host of the popular YouTube channel DadviceTV. James found my book easy to read and understand. It helped quiet the unnecessary fears that the medical establishment and social media had amplified around kidney disease. Patients who read my book and watched me on DadviceTV told me they felt less afraid, less confused, and more in control of their own health. Some discovered that they would likely never need dialysis. Many others learned they might not even have kidney disease at all. Their responses convinced me to write this book.

This book is for you whether you are in excellent health and want to stay that way, or managing conditions like type 2 diabetes, heart disease, or obesity and looking for what actually helps. Roughly one in three people in the developed world is living with at least one of these health challenges. A key message of this book is that how long you live and how well you age is largely within your control. The World Health Organization estimates that 40 to 60 percent of the leading causes of death and disability are shaped by lifestyle choices — choices that are in your hands.

The book speaks to a wide range of readers: the young high performer or biohacker in their 30s and 40s; the 45-to-65 group who are beginning to notice the signs of aging and want to remain active into their 80s and 90s; and the fast-growing population of adults over 65. Wherever you are in that spectrum, there is something here for you.

The book is organized in three sections. Section One covers the interventions with the greatest impact on lifespan and health span — the years of healthy, functional life. It begins with exercise—the single most powerful thing you can do for your health at any age, and something I personally practice every morning. From there, it addresses nutrition and the new generation of weight-loss medications; strategies to prevent heart attacks and strokes; a practical roadmap for maintaining brain function into old age; a guide for reversing type 2 diabetes through movement and diet; and a brief overview of the science of genetics, to show why your genes are not your destiny. The section closes with evidence-based strategies for reducing cancer risk.

Section Two takes a system-by-system tour of the aging body — muscles and joints, skin, hormones, eyes and ears, gut, kidneys, immune function, and lungs — explaining what changes are inevitable, which are preventable, and what the evidence says about managing each one.

Section Three opens with a deep dive into one of the most important and most overlooked factors in a long, good life:

mental health. From there, I examine the experimental therapies, supplements, and anti-aging interventions that have generated enormous excitement and, in many cases, enormous profits. I evaluate each one honestly. Some hold real promise. Most do not yet have the evidence to justify their cost or risk.

I close with a look at artificial intelligence and what it may mean for medicine in the years ahead—not as speculation, but as a realistic picture of a transformation already underway. Throughout every chapter, I have tried to keep one question in mind: what does the reader actually need to know? The result, I hope, is a book that respects your intelligence, your time, and your genuine desire to take control of your own health. The power to live longer and better is more within your reach than you may have imagined.

To make the book as useful as possible, every chapter is organized by subheading, and the Table of Contents lists every subheading so you can find any specific topic in seconds. I do recommend reading Section One in full — it covers the lifestyle interventions with the greatest impact on how long and how well you live, and the chapters build on each other in ways that are worth following in order. Section Two, which takes a system-by-system look at the aging body, is well suited to dipping in and out as your own health needs arise: if insomnia is a concern, Chapter 6 is where to look; if you are dealing with low back pain or sciatica, Chapter 10 addresses that directly; if you are experiencing a vision issue, Chapter 13 is the place to start. As you can see in the Table of Contents, I try to address the major health issues that you or your friends or family members may have now or develop in the future. Section Three's chapters on mental health, experimental therapies, and artificial intelligence can be read in any order. Think of this book less as something to read once and more as a reliable guide to return to.

Many readers will be reading this on behalf of an aging parent, partner, or family member. The information in this book applies as much to those caring for others as to those caring for themselves.

Table of Contents

Section One:

Lifestyle choices with the greatest impact.

"THE NINE CHAPTERS THAT follow cover the lifestyle choices with the most powerful, best-documented effects on how long you live and how healthy those years will be. These choices can add years to your life, slow the progression of chronic disease, and protect your brain, your heart, and your independence well into old age. The patients and friends who thrived into old age were rarely the ones with the best genes or the most money. They were the ones who understood what actually mattered and acted on it. Exercise comes first because nothing else comes close — not a single medication, supplement, or procedure matches what consistent movement does for the human body. From there, we move through diet and weight loss, the silent damage of atherosclerosis, the steps that protect brain function, the real possibility of reversing type 2 diabetes, and the evidence on cancer prevention. We end with genetics — not to discourage you, but to free you from the belief that your future is already written. It is not. The science in these chapters is settled enough to act on. My hope is that you will."

Chapter 1:

Exercise is the Modern "Fountain of Youth"

> *"Lack of activity destroys the good condition of every human being, while movement and methodical physical exercise save it and preserve it."*
>
> *– Plato*

IF EXERCISE WERE A pill, it would be the most prescribed medication in history—and the one with the fewest side effects. I have spent decades watching patients transform their health not through surgery or medication, but through the simple, transformative act of moving their bodies every day. The research is extraordinary: exercise touches virtually every system in the body, slows the aging process at the cellular level, and adds years—good years—to your life. I go to the gym every morning, alternating between weights and cardio, and I have seen firsthand what that commitment does over time. But you do not need a gym. Throughout this chapter, I will show you how to get the benefits of exercise wherever you are, whatever your starting point—and I will share the science that explains why it works.

Benefits of Exercise

The returns on exercise are remarkable. For every minute you invest, research suggests you get back up to seven minutes of additional lifespan—meaning consistent exercisers may live 3 to 7 years longer than their sedentary peers. But more time is not the only prize. Exercise lowers blood pressure, reduces LDL ("bad") cholesterol, and shrinks belly fat that drives heart disease and stroke. Combined with a healthy diet, it can manage—and in some cases reverse—type 2 diabetes. It stimulates the release of brain chemicals that lift mood and ease anxiety, and promotes neuroplasticity—the growth of new brain cells and new connections between them—which may be your best defense against Alzheimer's disease. Weight-bearing exercise builds bone density and fights sarcopenia (the age-related loss of muscle mass), while improving the balance that protects you from falls. It even lowers the risk of several cancers, decreases chronic pain, and deepens sleep. No medication on earth has this profile.

Understanding Exercise Research

Long-term animal studies—and a growing body of human research—reveal that exercise remodels virtually every tissue in the body. It strengthens the heart muscle and increases how much blood it pumps per minute, while training the nervous system to slow the heart rate at rest, making each beat more efficient. In muscle cells, exercise dramatically improves glucose uptake—essentially training your body to use sugar more effectively and lowering your diabetes risk. Resistance training builds muscle tissue that burns calories even while you sleep, which can help you maintain a healthy weight. Exercise also triggers the production of Brain-Derived Neurotrophic Factor (BDNF)—sometimes called “Miracle-Gro for the brain”—a protein directly linked to sharper memory, better concentration, and faster learning. It strengthens the immune system, extends the length of telomeres (the protective caps on your chromosomes that determine how fast your cells age), and even activates the cellular “cleanup crew” that removes damaged proteins before they cause harm (see Chapter 19).

Getting Started

The most important thing about starting an exercise habit is this: start smaller than you think you need to. Not a 45-minute gym session—a 10-minute walk. Not perfection—just showing up. I tell my patients: do not focus on how hard you work, focus on how consistently you show up. Three days a week is a great initial target. Once showing up feels automatic, the intensity will come naturally. Make it enjoyable—you might want to listen to podcasts or music, like I do. Many of my friends like to listen to audiobooks, explore new neighborhoods on foot, and go to Zumba classes, which make exercise more enjoyable. If you can find an exercise partner, do it. It is much harder to cancel on a friend than to cancel on yourself.

Setting Exercise Goals

Your long-term target is 150 minutes of moderate-intensity aerobic exercise per week—about 30 minutes on most days—

plus strength training two to three times a week. But that is a target, not a starting line. If you are currently doing nothing, even 10 minutes a day is a great start. For structured workout ideas, the Nerd Fitness program is an excellent, beginner-friendly resource.

Minimizing Risks of Exercise

For most people, beginning a moderate exercise program is far safer than remaining sedentary—but a few cautions are worth noting. If you have known heart disease, or are older and have not been active in years, check with your doctor before starting. Rare but serious cardiac events can occur in people with undiagnosed heart conditions who suddenly exert themselves vigorously. Beyond the heart, exercise in extreme heat raises the risk of dehydration and heat stroke, and extreme exertion can cause muscle breakdown severe enough to temporarily shut down the kidneys. The simple rules: do not push through pain, increase intensity gradually, and if you are unsure about technique, a single session with a certified trainer can save you months of injury. One more underappreciated risk: some people become compulsive about exercise, turning a healthy habit into a source of stress and burnout. More is not always better. Listen to your body.

Stretching

Stretching is a small investment that pays outsized dividends in injury prevention. A few minutes before a workout warms the muscles and prepares them for load; a few minutes afterward helps prevent stiffness and supports recovery. One important caveat: hold each stretch for 20–30 seconds, not longer. Holding a cold muscle in a sustained stretch for more than a minute can cause the very strain you are trying to prevent.

Cardio Exercises

The term "cardio," sometimes also referred to as aerobic exercise, refers to exercise that raises your heart rate and keeps it elevated for a sustained period, which can help improve the function of your heart, lungs, and blood vessels.

Walking

Hippocrates called it "man's best medicine," and two thousand years of science has yet to prove him wrong. Walking is the single most underrated form of exercise—free, low-risk, available to almost everyone, and backed by extraordinary evidence. A brisk daily walk of 30 to 60 minutes reduces the risk of cardiovascular death as effectively as running, with a fraction of the injury rate. Because it is weight-bearing, it maintains bone density in a way that swimming or cycling cannot. I have patients in their 80s who credit a daily walk with keeping them mobile, independent, and mentally sharp—and the research supports them. If you do nothing else after reading this chapter, walk.

Step Counts / Speed

If you use a fitness tracker, aim for 7,000 to 9,000 steps per day—that is where the evidence suggests the benefits plateau. But speed matters as much as distance: brisk walking reduces mortality risk by 30 percent compared to a slow stroll, and faster walkers show less age-related brain shrinkage. Over time, daily walking preserves mobility, reduces fall risk, and significantly lowers the chance of developing dementia.

Your Heart Rate

General movement—even gentle walking—is the foundation of reduced mortality risk. That said, once movement becomes a habit, adding intensity pays dividends. Picking up your pace until you are slightly breathless—what exercise scientists call "moderate intensity"—amplifies the cardiovascular and metabolic benefits significantly. Think of it as a dial you turn up gradually, not a switch you flip.

Strength Training

If cardio is the foundation, strength training is the structure built on top of it. People who combine strength training with cardio have a lower mortality risk than those who do cardio alone. The reason becomes clear when you understand what happens to muscle as we age: without regular resistance training, most adults lose 3 to 8 percent of their muscle mass per decade after 30. This is not cosmetic—it drives falls, fractures, metabolic decline, and loss of independence. Strength training builds denser bones, improves insulin sensitivity, and keeps you functionally capable well into old age. And you do not need a gym: push-ups, squats, lunges, and resistance bands are all highly effective. If you do have weights, aim for three sets of 8–12 repetitions per major muscle group, gradually increasing the load as it gets easier. The key word is "gradually."

Rowing for Strength and Cardio

Of all the exercise equipment I have tried over the years, the rowing machine remains my favorite recommendation—and the most underused piece of equipment in any gym. Rowing simultaneously trains the cardiovascular system and nearly every major muscle group: legs, core, back, arms. Studies show it delivers cardiovascular benefits equivalent to running, while the low impact is far gentler on the joints. There is also something almost meditative about the rhythm of rowing—it is one of the few exercises I find genuinely calming. I alternate rowing with targeted resistance machines on different days. If you are shopping for home equipment and have the space, I would put a rowing machine at the top of the list.

Improving Balance

Falls are the leading cause of injury-related death in adults over 65—and most of them are preventable. Balance training is the underappreciated tool that can change that statistic. Research shows it produces better functional outcomes than strength training alone. You do not need a special class: stand on one foot while you brush your teeth, practice heel-to-toe walking down a hallway, or try gentle yoga poses. Aim for 5 to 10 minutes, three times a week.

Movement Can Improve Mental Health

The mental health benefits of exercise are not a side effect—they are one of the primary effects. Vigorous exercise floods the bloodstream with endorphins (the source of the famous "runner's high"), but you do not need to run a 5K to feel the shift. Even a brisk 20-minute walk elevates endorphin levels. Exercise also increases endocannabinoids—neurotransmitters that bind to the same receptors as cannabis, generating feelings of calm and reducing anxiety without any of the downsides of smoking pot. Over time, regular movement literally remodels the brain's fear center (the amygdala), making it less reactive to stress. Perhaps most powerfully: for mild to moderate depression, exercise has been shown in multiple clinical trials to be as effective as psychotherapy and medication.

Exercise and Weight Loss

Let us dispel a stubborn myth: exercise alone is a poor weight-loss strategy. This is not an excuse to skip exercise—it is a fact about how the body works, and understanding it protects you from frustration. The brain, liver, and muscles each account for about 20 percent of your daily calorie burn. When you add exercise, your muscles may burn slightly more—but your brain or liver often compensates by burning slightly less, keeping the total roughly constant. On top of that, exercise makes many people hungry. A 30-minute run burns 250 to 400 calories; a post-run latte and muffin can easily cancel out those calories. And if you are doing strength training, you may actually gain weight initially as you build muscle, since muscle weighs more than fat. The solution is not to exercise less; it is to pair movement with mindful eating. Together, they work. Separately, neither is enough. Chapter 2 covers diet in detail.

Exercise Bursts Versus Any Movement

High-intensity interval training—HIIT—has become the fitness world's favorite buzzword, and for good reason: alternating short bursts of near-maximal effort with recovery periods delivers impressive results in less time. But here is what the HIIT hype can obscure: any movement is profoundly beneficial. Research shows that just three to four 1-minute bursts of vigorous activity scattered through the day significantly reduce mortality risk. Getting up and walking for 2 to 3 minutes every 30 minutes of sitting provides measurable long-term health benefits. Prolonged sitting is harmful to health, so try to engage in regular movement throughout the day. If you work from home or sit for long stretches, a standing desk is a great investment. My advice on HIIT: only add it once you are already exercising consistently. It is not a starting point—it is the next level. And always check with your doctor first, since it does carry a higher injury risk, particularly for those returning to exercise after a long break.

Conclusion

Plato understood something two millennia ago that we now have the science to prove: movement is not optional. It is the most powerful medicine available to you—free, accessible, and effective against almost every major cause of aging and death. It adds years to your life and life to your years. Start with a walk. Find a partner. Put on a podcast. Show up three days a week until showing up feels like breathing—natural, automatic, and missed when it is gone. Work toward 150 minutes of moderate aerobic activity weekly, in addition to strength training at least two to three times a week. Focus on a diet and exercise routine you can consistently maintain. Be like many of my gym friends and daily walker friends who in their 70s, 80s, and 90s remain active, healthy, and vibrant by tapping into the exercise "Fountain of Youth."

Chapter 2:

Your Weight, Diet, and Weight Loss Medications

IF YOU HAVE EVER lost weight only to gain it back—and felt like you somehow failed—this chapter is for you. The science of weight, diet, and metabolism is more nuanced than most people realize, and understanding it is the first step toward stopping the cycle. We will look at why diets so often disappoint in the long run, how your brain and gut actively resist weight loss, and what you can do that actually works. We will cover the Mediterranean diet—the most evidence-based eating pattern—the serious harms of ultra-processed foods, and the remarkable new class of GLP-1 weight loss medications that are transforming what is possible for people struggling with obesity.

Why Dieting Often Fails

Here is a fact that should change how you think about your dieting history: more than 80 percent of people who lose weight regain it within three to five years. That is not a character flaw; it is your biology. Your body defends a natural weight "set point" the way a thermostat defends a temperature—and when you lose weight, it fights back. Ghrelin, the hormone that makes you hungry, surges, and leptin, the hormone that tells you are full, drops. Your metabolism quietly adjusts so that your body burns fewer calories at your lower weight. It seems as though the deck is stacked against you— every time you try to lose weight.

Emerging research is beginning to identify distinct subtypes of weight gain: the "hungry brain," where you simply need more calories to feel satisfied than most people do; the "hungry gut," where hunger returns surprisingly quickly after eating; and emotional eating, where food becomes a primary tool for managing stress, grief, or boredom. Future programs will increasingly target these patterns individually. The most effective strategy remains gradual weight loss—about 1 to 2 pounds per week—combined with durable changes to both eating habits and physical activity. Crash diets produce crash results.

Who is Considered Obese?

About 42 percent of American adults are currently classified as obese—defined as a Body Mass Index (BMI) over 30, calculated by dividing weight in kilograms by height in meters squared. Alarmingly, nearly 20 percent of U.S. children are also obese. But BMI is an imperfect tool. It does not distinguish between muscle and fat, so a muscular athlete may register as "obese" while a sedentary person with dangerous levels of visceral (belly) fat may land in the "normal" range. Medical thinking has evolved. Obesity is now increasingly classified as a chronic disease rather than a personal failing. The distinction between "preclinical" obesity (excess fat without health consequences yet) and "clinical" obesity (excess fat actively driving disease—heart disease, liver damage, type 2 diabetes) matters not only medically but practically, since a clinical obesity classification affects insurance eligibility for weight loss medications in the United States.

Mindful Eating

Your brain is at the center of your weight, not your willpower. One of the most practical tools available is mindful eating—a set of habits that work with your biology rather than against it. Eat slowly and drink water between bites; it takes about 20 minutes for fullness signals to reach your brain. If you eat fast you will consistently overshoot this brain signal. Stop eating when you feel about 80 percent full—satisfied, not stuffed. Notice when you are reaching for food out of boredom or stress rather than genuine hunger. Aim for three regular meals and one or two small snacks per day; going too long without eating tends to produce the kind of extreme hunger that overrides all good intentions. The goal is not perfection—it is finding an eating pattern you can actually sustain for years, not weeks.

Benefits and Harms From What We Eat

The Mediterranean Diet

Of all the eating patterns studied in modern medicine, the Mediterranean diet has the strongest and most consistent evidence behind it. Built around whole grains, legumes (beans), nuts, fish, olive oil, fruits, and vegetables—with modest amounts of dairy and poultry and very little red meat—it does far more than manage weight. Large, well-designed trials show it improves insulin sensitivity, lowers chronic inflammation, protects brain health, and is associated with a 20 percent reduction in the risk of premature death. That protection spans cancer, heart disease, type 2 diabetes, and Alzheimer's. One key reason it works long-term: it does not demand that you eliminate entire food groups. Unlike the keto diet, which restricts carbohydrates so severely that long-term adherence is difficult and the high saturated fat content raises its own concerns, the Mediterranean diet is something most people can eat for the rest of their lives—and want to. For recipes, The Mediterranean Dish, Mediterranean Living, Eating Well, and Skinnytaste are all excellent starting points.

The Importance of Fiber

Fiber may be the single most underappreciated nutrient in the diet. The Mediterranean diet delivers fiber in abundance, and the benefits are wide-ranging. Fiber feeds the gut microbiome—the trillions of microbes living in your intestine—which respond by producing anti-inflammatory compounds that reduce the risk of chronic disease throughout the body. Fiber also slows glucose absorption, blunting blood sugar spikes that drive diabetes and heart disease, while lowering LDL cholesterol and blood pressure. Fiber also helps prevent constipation and dramatically reduces the risk of colorectal cancer, diverticulitis, hemorrhoids, and inflammatory bowel disease. And practically, it keeps you fuller longer—which means less mindless snacking. A fiber-rich diet is simply a whole-food diet: whole grains, fruits, vegetables, beans, and nuts. For specific high-fiber recipe ideas, Delish's 20 high-fiber recipes, The Real Food Dietitians' high-fiber dinners, and the Mayo Clinic's high-fiber foods list are all worth bookmarking.

Ultra-Processed Foods

At the opposite end of the dietary spectrum from the Mediterranean style diet sit ultra-processed foods—and the contrast in health outcomes is stark. A landmark study drawing on data from nearly 10 million people found what researchers called "convincing evidence" linking high UPF intake to 32 separate health problems, including a 50 percent increased risk of death from cardiovascular disease, a comparable increase in anxiety and mental health disorders, and a 20 percent higher risk of death from any cause.

Ultra-processed foods now account for more than half of all calories consumed by U.S. adults and children—and the health toll is visible in our obesity, diabetes, and depression rates. The defining feature of a UPF is not that it has been cooked or preserved, but that it has been fundamentally transformed and loaded with ingredients you would not find in a home kitchen: artificial flavors, emulsifiers, colorings, and preservatives designed to maximize palatability and shelf life. Fresh fruit is not processed. Canned tuna is minimally processed. A bag of flavored chips engineered to be impossible to stop eating is ultra-processed—and it activates the brain's reward center in ways that undermine normal hunger regulation. Watch for misleading labels: "all-natural," "low-calorie," and "cholesterol-free" are marketing terms, not health certifications. The simplest rule: if the ingredient list is long and contains words you do not recognize, put it back. Apps like Fooducate or MyNetDiary can help you evaluate specific products quickly.

What Are "Healthy Fats"?

For decades, dietary fat was treated as a single villain—a mistake that sent millions of people toward low-fat processed foods that were, in many cases, worse for their health. The science is now clear: fat is not the problem. The type of fat is. Healthy unsaturated fats—found in olive oil, avocados, and nuts—are anti-inflammatory and protective of heart and brain health. Omega-3 fatty acids specifically—found in fatty fish like salmon and mackerel, as well as walnuts and flaxseed—provide particularly strong cardiovascular and brain benefits. Trans fats, by contrast, are genuinely dangerous: they raise LDL ("bad") cholesterol, lower HDL ("good") cholesterol, and significantly increase the risk of heart disease and stroke. Trans fats are created when liquid oils are partially hydrogenated—a process used to extend shelf life in fried fast foods, pastries, pizza dough, donuts, cookies, and crackers. The American Heart Association emphasizes replacing saturated and trans fats with unsaturated fats, rather than targeting a specific percentage of daily calories from fat—and recommends zero tolerance for trans fats.

Restrict Dietary Alcohol

For years, many of us went along with the "a glass of red wine is good for you" narrative. Recent evidence has strongly disputed this advice. A study of nearly 5 million people found that moderate drinking offered no meaningful protection against death compared to abstaining—and that women who consumed more than two drinks daily and men who exceeded three faced significantly higher mortality risk. This matters because alcohol is not a neutral substance. It raises blood pressure, inflames the pancreas (sometimes fatally, in the case of pancreatitis), scars the liver (cirrhosis), causes gastrointestinal bleeding, and contributes to fluid accumulation in the abdomen (ascites). In later chapters I will explain in more detail how it accelerates cognitive decline and meaningfully raises cancer risk. Beyond the physical effects: alcohol disrupts sleep architecture, worsens anxiety and depression, and impairs the judgment and motor control that protect you from falls and accidents. And for those with a family history of alcohol use disorder or mental illness, the addiction risk is substantially elevated. I am not suggesting everyone must abstain—but the evidence no longer supports drinking for health.

Dietary Supplements

The supplement industry generates over $50 billion a year in the United States, largely on the back of studies too small and too short to mean much—and marketing designed to exploit hope. For healthy people eating a reasonably balanced diet, the evidence is consistently unimpressive. For example, a study of 400000 healthy adults followed over 20 years confirmed that multivitamin use was not associated with a lower risk of death. Another study found that Beta-carotene supplements may actually increase lung cancer risk in smokers.

Whole foods deliver nutrients in complex combinations that supplements simply cannot replicate, and excess water-soluble vitamins (vitamin C and B complex) are typically excreted in urine anyway. What supplements can do is cause harm: unlike prescription drugs, they are not FDA-approved for safety or efficacy, may contain contaminants including heavy metals and pesticides, and can interact with medications in ways that reduce drug effectiveness or cause toxicity. There are genuine exceptions—specific deficiencies, specific medical conditions—and your doctor can tell you if you are one of them. But "just in case" supplementation is not the same as good nutrition.

Weight Loss Medications

For most of medical history, weight loss drug effects were modest at best—producing average losses of 2 to 10 percent of body weight. The GLP-1 receptor agonists have changed the prescription weight loss options, fundamentally. These medications mimic GLP-1, a hormone naturally released by your gut after eating that signals the brain to reduce appetite. Originally developed for type 2 diabetes, they turned out to produce significant amounts of weight loss that previous drugs could not approach. A newer class of drugs targets a second gut hormone called GIP (glucose-dependent insulinotropic polypeptide), amplifying the effect further. Together, these drugs can produce weight loss of 15 to 20 percent of body weight—territory previously achievable only through bariatric surgery (see Chapter 7). They work by stimulating insulin release when blood sugar rises, suppressing glucagon (a hormone that raises blood sugar), and slowing stomach emptying so you feel full longer.

Two leading drugs are semaglutide, sold as Wegovy for weight loss and Ozempic at a lower dose for diabetes; and tirzepatide, sold as Zepbound for obesity and Mounjaro for diabetes. Tirzepatide targets both GLP-1 and GIP receptors, producing a stronger response with somewhat fewer gastrointestinal side effects than semaglutide. Both are injected once weekly. Most patients notice reduced appetite within the first two to four weeks; by twelve weeks of gradually increasing doses, average body weight has typically declined by 6 to 8 percent. The critical caveat: when the medication is stopped, most of the lost weight returns within a year. These are not cure-and-done treatments—they are long-term medications, much like blood pressure drugs. For that reason, I always advise combining them with a Mediterranean diet and the exercise habits described in the previous chapter. The medication provides a window of opportunity; what you do with that opportunity determines the lasting result.

Downsides of GLP-1 Medications

These medications are genuinely powerful, and they come with real downsides worth knowing before you start. Nausea, vomiting, diarrhea, and abdominal discomfort are common, particularly in the early weeks of treatment—and they are unpleasant enough that roughly half of all patients discontinue within a year. Rapid weight loss can trigger gallstones. Fat loss in the face (widely nicknamed "Ozempic face") can produce a gaunt, aged appearance that some patients find distressing. And while the overall safety profile appears favorable based on current data, these are still relatively new drugs and long-term data—covering decades of use—do not yet exist. Proceed with realistic expectations and close medical supervision.

Older Adults and GLP-1 Drugs

I want to address older adults specifically, because the risk-benefit calculation for GLP-1 drugs shifts meaningfully with age. Adults over 65 are considerably more susceptible to persistent nausea, vomiting, and diarrhea—and in seniors, these symptoms can rapidly produce dangerous dehydration, low blood pressure and a decline in kidney function. In addition to the harms of dehydration, rapid weight loss in older adults pulls as much as 25 to 40 percent of that lost weight from muscle and bone rather than fat. That is a significant problem. Loss of muscle mass and bone density leads to thin bones (osteoporosis—see Chapter 10), fractures, reduced mobility, and a higher risk of falls—some of the very outcomes we most want to prevent in aging. Many of my older patients stop the medication when they or their physicians notice declining strength or mobility, and that is often the right call. If you are over 65 and considering these drugs, increasing protein intake and committing to resistance training are not optional add-ons—they are essential countermeasures. And it is worth asking honestly whether the trade-offs—including the loss of one of life's genuine pleasures, the social and emotional dimension of meals—is worth it for you.

Cost of Weight Loss Drugs

Cost is a real barrier. These are among the most expensive

medications in common use, and insurance coverage is inconsistent. The encouraging news: Medicare and Medicaid now cover GLP-1 drugs for qualifying patients in the U.S. Generic versions are still roughly a decade away for the injected forms. In the meantime, some compounding pharmacies offer lower-cost versions—but these are not FDA-approved, and their safety, potency, and purity cannot be guaranteed. I would caution strongly against compounded versions without a thorough discussion with your physician.

Oral GLP-1 Drugs

The next frontier is pills. Oral semaglutide—essentially the Wegovy molecule in tablet form—is already available, though it requires strict dosing instructions: empty stomach, small sip of water, 30-minute wait before eating. Competing oral forms of the drug, without the dosing requirements of oral semaglutide are in development and companies are racing to market with their own versions. Competition is expected to push monthly costs as low as $150 a month, dramatically broadening access. Once-monthly injectable formulations are also in development. There will likely be cheaper formulations with less side effects in the future.

Potential Benefits of Weight Loss

The health benefits of meaningful weight loss extend well beyond the obvious. For patients with joint pain, shedding excess weight removes mechanical load from knees, hips, and spine—often delaying or eliminating the need for joint replacement surgery, and reducing complications if surgery becomes necessary. Gastrointestinal reflux (GERD - see Chapter 14) and sleep apnea frequently improve or resolve with weight loss. Blood pressure may normalize. Blood sugar control improves dramatically—and in some patients who combine weight loss with sustained exercise, type 2 diabetes may go into remission (see Chapter 7). These are major quality-of-life improvements.

Two conditions particularly worth understanding are metabolic syndrome and MASLD. Metabolic syndrome is a cluster of problems—excess abdominal fat, elevated blood sugar, high blood pressure, and high LDL cholesterol—that together dramatically increase the risk of heart disease, diabetes, and stroke. MASLD (metabolic dysfunction-associated steatosis liver disease) is a related condition in which fat accumulates in the liver, causing inflammation and, in a subset of patients, progressing to cirrhosis and liver cancer. Both sound alarming, but both are highly responsive to lifestyle change. Healthier eating, more physical activity, and even modest weight loss—as little as 5 to 10 percent—can reverse or significantly reduce both conditions.

Does Weight Loss Increase Longevity?

Intentional, sustained weight loss—especially when it reverses metabolic syndrome or MASLD—can meaningfully extend life. Even a 5 to 10 percent reduction in body weight lowers systolic blood pressure, fasting blood glucose, and LDL cholesterol, each of which independently reduces the risk of heart attack and stroke. At the extreme end, severe obesity carries mortality risks comparable to lifelong smoking. On the other hand, being overweight does not automatically mean poor health outcomes, and fixating on weight can sometimes lead us to miss what actually matters. A physically active person classified as overweight by BMI often has far better health outcomes than a sedentary person in the "normal" weight range. For older adults especially, the risks of aggressive weight loss—muscle wasting, bone loss, falls, fractures, hospitalizations—can outweigh the benefits. And for people who are not obese—particularly older adults—intentional weight loss may actually shorten rather than extend life expectancy. Another important distinction: intentional weight loss (pursued deliberately) has different health implications than unintentional weight loss, which is often a warning sign of underlying disease—cancer, organ failure—and is associated with shorter survival. If you are losing weight without trying, see your doctor.

Conclusion

The goal of this chapter is to free you from obsessing over the number on the scale, help you eat well, move consistently, and understand the medications available when those strategies are not enough on their own. Your weight is not simply a matter of discipline. It is the combination of your biology, environment, habits and hormones. Dieting alone rarely works long-term because your body fights back. What does work is a durable shift toward whole foods, especially a Mediterranean-style eating pattern, combined with regular physical activity and a reduction in ultra-processed foods. For those with obesity-related health complications, GLP-1 medications now offer a genuine medical intervention—but they work best, and last longest, when paired with the lifestyle changes that keep the weight from returning. The number on the scale is one data point. How you feel, move, sleep, and function are better things to focus on.

Chapter 3:

Slowing Atherosclerosis: A Key to Lifespan and Health Span

HEART DISEASE KILLS MORE people in high-income countries than any other cause—and much of that death is preventable. The culprit, in most cases, is atherosclerosis: the slow, decades-long buildup of fatty plaque inside artery walls that gradually narrows vessels until blood flow is compromised, or until a plaque ruptures and triggers a clot. Heart attacks, strokes, and peripheral artery disease together account for more than one-third of deaths in developed nations. The good news is that atherosclerosis is not inevitable, and its progression can be meaningfully slowed. Exercise and diet—covered in the previous two chapters—are foundational. This chapter adds two more targets that are just as critical: getting your systolic blood pressure below 120 and your LDL ("bad") cholesterol below 70. We will also address smoking, which remains among the most powerful accelerants of vascular disease, and clarify the evidence on daily aspirin.

What is Atherosclerosis?

Atherosclerosis is not a disease of old age—it begins in childhood. When excess LDL cholesterol circulates in the blood, it accumulates beneath the inner lining of artery walls, triggering inflammation. The body dispatches white blood cells to contain the damage, but the result is a growing mass of cholesterol-laden cells—plaque—encased in a fibrous cap. For years or decades, this plaque sits silently, narrowing the vessel and reducing blood flow. The danger escalates when the fibrous cap ruptures: the body responds by forming a clot, and if that clot is large enough to block the artery completely, the tissue downstream dies. In the heart, that is a heart attack; in the brain, a stroke; in the legs, it can progress to amputation. The risk factors that accelerate this process—high LDL, high blood pressure, diabetes, obesity, chronic kidney disease—are all increasingly common. The interventions that slow it—a Mediterranean diet, regular exercise, and targeted medications—are all available to you now.

Elevated Blood Pressure and Atherosclerosis

High blood pressure is the single most powerful and prevalent driver of atherosclerosis-related deaths. It accelerates plaque formation, damages artery walls, and dramatically increases the risk of heart attack, stroke, and kidney failure—often without producing a single symptom until the damage is done. That is why it has earned the name "silent killer." The only way to know your blood pressure number is to measure it. A drop of 10 mmHg in systolic blood pressure (the top number) translates to roughly a 20 percent reduction in the risk of major cardiovascular events. That is an extraordinary return on a modest change.

How to Measure Blood Pressure

Most people have had their blood pressure measured inaccurately at some point—taken too quickly, in the wrong position, on a cuff that did not fit properly. Inaccurate readings lead to either under-treatment (missing a real problem) or over-treatment (medicating normal values). I recommend that all my patients own an affordable automatic blood pressure monitor, one that displays both systolic and diastolic readings along with heart rate. Home measurement, done correctly, tells you far more than an isolated office reading.

Technique matters. Sit quietly for at least five minutes before measuring—no conversation, no phone. Your arm should rest at heart level, supported, with your back straight and feet flat on the floor. Make sure that the cuff wraps around your upper arm at least one and a quarter times. Take at least two readings spaced five minutes apart and record both. Share your home blood pressure recordings with your provider since they may be very different than a single in-office measurement taken under stress.

When to Check Blood Pressure

Monitoring your blood pressure at home between visits is one of the most effective things you can do for your cardiovascular health (cardio refers to heart, vascular refers to arteries and veins). Studies show that patients who actively track and share their blood pressure readings achieve significantly better control than those who rely on office visits alone. Check it anytime you feel dizzy or weak, especially when standing, as that can signal overtreatment. I have experienced this personally: my own blood pressure dropped too low on my usual medication, and I had to adjust. If your systolic reading falls below 90 to 100, contact your provider about temporarily holding your medication until it rises above 110. Overtreatment—pushing blood pressure too low—can reduce critical blood flow to the heart, brain, and kidneys.

Challenges in Diagnosing High Blood Pressure

Home readings are essential partly because of a well-documented phenomenon called "white coat hypertension"—blood pressure that spikes in the doctor's office due to anxiety. This is a common phenomenon, which can lead to adding unnecessary blood pressure medication. Your home readings give a more accurate assessment your 24 hour blood pressure levels than any single measurement.

While both numbers matter, systolic blood pressure is the primary target for preventing cardiovascular disease. In older adults, arteries naturally stiffen with age, which tends to push systolic blood pressure up while diastolic pressure stays the same or drops. This pattern—called isolated systolic hypertension—is extremely common. A diastolic reading above 90 may warrant treatment, but pushing it below 80 generally provides no additional benefit—and a diastolic below 60 can actually reduce blood flow to the heart, potentially triggering chest pain.

Goal Blood Pressure — Less Than 120 Systolic

The target for blood pressure has changed dramatically

over the past two decades—and for good reason. A systolic of 160 was once considered acceptable for older adults; we now know that cardiovascular risk begins rising meaningfully above 130 systolic regardless of a patient's age. Getting systolic blood pressure below 120 reduces the risk of heart attacks, heart failure, stroke, chronic kidney disease, and cognitive decline—all of which become more common with age. For the small subset of older patients who are frail, have multiple medical conditions, or experience significant dizziness when standing, a target of 130 to 140 systolic is a reasonable compromise. For everyone else, lower is better.

The relationship between systolic blood pressure and mortality is direct and linear: the higher it goes, the greater the risk. Current classifications place anything below 120/80 as normal; 120–129 as elevated; 130–139/80–89 as Stage 1 hypertension; and 140/90 or above as Stage 2. For many patients, a 10 to 20 percent reduction in weight, reduced salt intake, and regular exercise can bring blood pressure into target range without medication. But if systolic remains above 130 despite lifestyle changes, medication is appropriate—and most patients will ultimately need two or more drugs to reach their goal.

Causes of Poor Blood Pressure Control

Poor blood pressure control usually has a specific, identifiable cause—and the most common one is medication confusion. I always ask patients to bring every medication they take to their appointment, including supplements and over-the-counter drugs. Ideally, blood pressure medications should be taken once or at most twice daily; I take mine at night and at the same time every day—consistency matters more than which time you choose. If blood pressure remains difficult to control, adding a diuretic like hydrochlorothiazide (HCTZ) often helps. Common culprits that raise blood pressure include cocaine and stimulant medications like Adderall, heavy alcohol use, and a high-salt diet.

Most patients with hypertension have so called essential/primary hypertension- with no known cause. All patients with hypertension should have a kidney function and urine protein test, since kidney disease is one of the commonest causes of secondary hypertension (see Chapter 15). Other secondary causes include adrenal hormone imbalances which are associated with a low blood potassium level, and narrowing of the kidney arteries (renal artery stenosis). These secondary causes are worth investigating in patients whose blood pressure remains difficult to control despite adequate medication.

Which Blood Pressure Medications Are Best?

My standard approach to blood pressure medications is to start with an ACE inhibitor-ACE with names ending in "-pril": lisinopril, enalapril, benazepril or an angiotensin receptor blocker-ARB, with names ending in "-tan": losartan, valsartan. These medications are well-tolerated, inexpensive, and offer additional protection for the kidneys and heart that goes beyond blood pressure lowering alone—making them especially valuable for patients with chronic kidney disease, diabetes, or heart failure. If an ACE inhibitor causes a persistent cough (a common side effect), switching to an ARB usually resolves the problem. Many ACE and ARB formulations come combined with a diuretic like hydrochlorothiazide in a single pill, which simplifies the regimen. When either an ACE or an ARB (it can be dangerous to use both classes together) are at their maximum dose and blood pressure remains elevated, I add a long-acting calcium channel blocker—amlodipine is my usual next choice.

Blood Pressure Drugs for Specific Situations

Other classes of blood pressure medications serve specific situations well. Beta blockers—like atenolol or metoprolol—significantly reduce mortality after a heart attack and are the standard of care for heart failure patients, typically prescribed lifelong. Men with both hypertension and an enlarged prostate may benefit from alpha blockers like terazosin, which address both problems, though the risk of blood pressure dropping when standing requires attention. For patients with truly resistant hypertension, minoxidil is a powerful option. And for hypertensive patients with a rapid resting heart rate, the calcium channel blockers diltiazem or verapamil can address both problems at once.

Cholesterol — Understanding HDL and LDL

Cholesterol medicine has a frustrating recent history of chasing the wrong target. For years, the assumption was that raising HDL ("good") cholesterol would protect the heart—mirroring the observation that people with naturally high HDL tend to have less heart disease. Several drugs raise HDL but they did essentially nothing for outcomes. Niacin (vitamin B3), which raises HDL substantially, not only failed to reduce heart disease deaths but was linked to serious infections, bleeding, and gastrointestinal complications. While a low HDL may still be a marker of cardiovascular risk, elevating HDL does not decrease atherosclerosis related deaths. What genuinely moves the needle is lowering LDL. Statins—which block cholesterol production in the liver and dramatically increase the liver's ability to clear LDL from the bloodstream—are among the most rigorously tested drugs in the history of medicine. Their ability to reduce heart attacks and strokes is not in dispute.

Target LDL Below 70

LDL targets have moved aggressively downward as the evidence has accumulated. A level below 160 was once considered acceptable; current guidelines recommend below 70 for most patients, and below 50 for those at highest risk—people with existing heart disease, kidney disease, or diabetes. Emerging trials are now examining whether pushing LDL below 20 mg/dL might provide even greater protection. The trend is consistent: lower LDL means fewer heart attacks and strokes, with no evidence of a floor below which the benefit disappears.

Most patients can reach their LDL target with the right statin at the right dose. If you are not hitting your goal, ask your provider about increasing your dose or switching to a more potent statin—atorvastatin and rosuvastatin are both highly effective and inexpensive in generic form. Ezetimibe, another low-cost option, blocks LDL absorption in the gut and pairs well with statins. For patients at the highest cardiovascular risk who still cannot reach target despite maximum therapy, PCSK9 inhibitors—evolocumab and alirocumab—are highly effective but expensive; insurers typically require documentation that simpler options have been tried and failed.

Atherosclerotic Plaque Instability

One of the most important and counterintuitive insights in cardiovascular medicine is that the size of a plaque matters less than its stability. Plaques do not kill people by slowly suffocating blood flow; they kill people by rupturing suddenly and triggering a clot. Soft, lipid-rich, inflamed plaques rupture. Hard, calcified, stable plaques do not—or at least, far less often. High-dose statins work in part by shrinking the lipid core of plaques and reducing their inflammation, making them more stable. As plaques stabilize on statin therapy, they often accumulate more calcium—which can appear alarming on a coronary calcium scan. Do not be misled: this "calcification paradox" is a sign of improvement, not deterioration. For patients already on statin therapy, what matters is plaque composition and stability, not the calcium score alone (see Chapter 4). GLP-1 receptor agonists may also stabilize plaque, which may help explain why they reduce heart attacks in patients with type 2 diabetes—though formal plaque stability studies are still pending.

Should You Take a Baby Aspirin Every Day?

The question of daily low-dose aspirin is one I am asked constantly, and the answer depends entirely on your situation.

Aspirin prevents clots from forming on ruptured plaques—which makes it powerful when you need it and risky when you do not. For secondary prevention—patients who have already had a heart attack, stroke, stent, or bypass, or who have ongoing chest pain from heart disease—daily baby aspirin (75 to 162 mg) can be lifesaving. For primary prevention—people trying to prevent a first cardiovascular event—the picture is more nuanced. Adults aged 40 to 60 with high cardiovascular risk and low bleeding risk may benefit from low-dose aspirin. But for those 60 and older, the bleeding risk in the brain and gastrointestinal tract may well outweigh the cardiovascular benefit. Talk to your doctor—this is genuinely an individual decision.

Atherosclerosis of the Aorta and Peripheral Arteries

Atherosclerosis does not confine itself to the heart and brain. In the legs, it causes peripheral artery disease, which typically presents as claudication—a cramping pain in the calf or thigh that comes on with walking and eases with rest. In severe cases, it produces wounds that will not heal and, ultimately, amputation. In the main artery of the abdomen (the aorta), the same process can create an abdominal aortic aneurysm (AAA)—a dangerous bulging of the vessel wall that can rupture catastrophically without warning. Men between 65 and 75 who have ever smoked, or who have a family history of AAA, should have a one-time ultrasound screening for this condition. It is a simple, painless test that can genuinely save a life.

Smoking and Atherosclerosis

If there is a single modifiable risk factor that most dramatically accelerates every form of vascular disease, it is smoking. Smokers represent the vast majority of peripheral artery disease cases, and their disease progresses to a need for limb amputation far faster than in non-smokers. Smoking is the strongest single predictor of abdominal aortic aneurysm development and rupture. For coronary artery disease, peripheral artery disease, and stroke, smoking consistently ranks among the top three risk factors alongside hypertension and high cholesterol. The mechanisms are direct: smoking raises LDL, lowers HDL, and dramatically increases the tendency of blood to clot on vulnerable plaques—a perfect storm for heart attacks and strokes.

How to Quit Smoking

Quitting smoking is hard—but the benefits begin almost immediately, and the risk of heart attack and stroke starts declining within weeks of stopping. Several evidence-based tools can help. Nicotine replacement therapy (NRT: patches, gum, lozenges) reduces withdrawal by delivering nicotine without the toxic combustion products of cigarettes. Varenicline (Chantix) targets nicotine receptors in the brain directly and is more effective than NRT alone, though it is more expensive. Vaping and e-cigarettes can help reduce intake gradually and are probably less harmful than cigarettes (which set an extremely low bar), but carry their own lung risks and have become a serious public health problem by hooking a new generation of non-smokers, particularly teenagers. Smokefree.gov offers free, personalized quit plans, and many insurance plans cover cessation medications and counseling. Use every tool available. The benefits of stopping—on your arteries, your lungs, your cancer risk, and your longevity—are among the most dramatic in all of medicine.

Conclusion

Atherosclerosis is not an inevitable consequence of aging—it is a modifiable process that responds to the choices you make every day. The four most powerful levers you have are: do not smoke (or stop if you do), get your blood pressure below 120 systolic, get your LDL below 70, and eat and exercise as described in the previous two chapters. Together, these interventions can dramatically reduce your risk of the heart attacks, strokes, and amputations that kill or disable more people in high-income countries than any other cause. The science is clear. The rest is up to you.

Chapter 4:

Age-Related Heart Diseases

HEART DISEASE KILLS ONE in three people worldwide. Coronary artery disease (CAD) alone—the progressive narrowing of the arteries that supply the heart muscle—accounts for roughly 40 to 45 percent of all cardiovascular deaths. In this chapter, we look at how your heart and blood vessels change with age, who should be screened for heart disease and with what tests, and—critically—what to do if you think you are having a heart attack. Remember: "time is muscle." We will also examine the evidence on stents (which are performed far more often than necessary), when bypass surgery may be necessary, and how to manage heart failure and atrial fibrillation, which become more prevalent with age.

Your Heart and Blood Vessels as You Age

The aging heart and blood vessels change in predictable ways. The heart muscle tends to thicken and stiffen, reducing its ability to relax and fill efficiently between beats. The ejection fraction (EF)—the percentage of blood pumped out with each beat—may decline from the normal 60 percent toward 40 percent or below. Artery walls stiffen and lose elasticity, driving up systolic blood pressure and making the heart work harder with every beat. Heart valves may become calcified and less pliable over time. The electrical system of the heart loses cells, which can lead to slow heart rates and irregular rhythms, including atrial fibrillation. Atherosclerosis—which began in childhood and has been progressing silently ever since—continues to narrow the coronary arteries. These changes are gradual and often invisible, which is precisely what makes them dangerous.

Coronary Artery Disease

The coronary arteries are the vessels that supply the heart muscle itself—a network that wraps around the outside of the heart and penetrates its walls. CAD develops when these arteries are progressively narrowed by atherosclerotic plaque (see Chapter 3). For years or decades, this process is completely silent—no symptoms, no warning. Then comes the event. Sometimes a plaque cracks or ruptures, triggering the body to form a clot at the site. If the clot is large enough to block the artery entirely, blood flow stops. The heart muscle downstream begins to die within minutes—this is a heart attack. For many people, CAD announces itself not with chest pain but with the heart attack itself. Which is why understanding the warning signs—and acting on them immediately—can be the difference between life and death.

Symptoms of Blocked Arteries to the Heart

At rest, even a significantly narrowed artery may deliver enough blood to the heart. But when you climb stairs, rush for a bus, or experience sudden emotional stress, the heart's oxygen demand surges—and a narrowed artery cannot keep up. The result is chest pain or pressure (angina), or in the worst case, a heart attack. While some heart attacks occur suddenly, many begin with mild discomfort. The cardinal warning sign is discomfort in the center of the chest lasting more than a few minutes, or that comes and goes. It may feel like pressure, squeezing, fullness, tightness, or frank pain. Pain or discomfort may radiate to the arms, back, neck, jaw, or stomach. Shortness of breath, cold sweats, nausea, and lightheadedness are other common features. If you experience these symptoms: call 911. Do not wait to see if it passes. Do not drive yourself. Every minute matters.

Signs of a Heart Attack in Women

Women are more likely than men to present with atypical symptoms—which is one reason their heart attacks are more often missed or delayed. While chest pain occurs in women too, they are more likely to experience shortness of breath, nausea, vomiting, unusual fatigue, and pain in the back or jaw rather than the classic crushing chest pressure. If something feels wrong, trust that instinct and call for help. Heart disease kills more women than any other condition.

What to Do if You Think You Are Having a Heart Attack

If you suspect a heart attack—call 911 immediately. This is the most important sentence in this chapter. Medical associations worldwide are aligned on this point: do not wait to see if symptoms resolve. The phrase "time is muscle" exists because that is exactly how the biology works—the heart muscle begins dying within 20 to 30 minutes of a complete blockage, and every additional minute of delay means more irreversible damage and a worse long-term outcome.

Do not drive yourself to the hospital. It wastes time—paramedics can begin treatment in the ambulance, before you arrive—and it puts you and others at serious risk if you lose consciousness behind the wheel. Let emergency services come to you.

Heart Attack Treatment

After calling 911 you should chew four 81 mg baby aspirin or chew one regular (325 mg) aspirin. Aspirin reduces clotting and can limit the extent of heart muscle damage. If there is a suspicion of a stomach ulcer, GI bleed, symptoms of a stroke (see Chapter 5) or aspirin allergy, taking aspirin may be harmful.

The definitive treatment is to open the blocked artery as fast as possible. The gold standard is balloon angioplasty—inflating a tiny balloon inside the blocked vessel to restore flow—typically followed immediately by placement of a stent to keep the artery open. This must happen within 90 to 120 minutes of symptom onset to salvage the maximum amount of heart muscle. When a catheterization lab is not immediately available—because the nearest capable hospital is too far away—intravenous clot-busting drugs (thrombolytics) can be given as a bridge until the patient can be transferred. Time is the variable that determines everything.

Cough CPR?

A dangerous myth circulates online claiming that "cough CPR"—deep breaths followed by forceful coughing—can stop a heart attack or restore a normal heart rhythm. It cannot. This technique has no evidence behind it and, worse, it can delay the one action that actually matters: calling for emergency help. Do not cough. Call 911.

How to Diagnose Coronary Artery Disease

Coronary Artery Calcium Scan

A coronary artery calcium (CAC) scan uses CT imaging to detect calcium deposits in the coronary arteries—a proxy for the total amount of atherosclerotic plaque present. A CAC score of zero is reassuring: it significantly reduces the likelihood of a near-term cardiac event. However, the test has important limitations. It only detects calcified plaque, not the soft, non-calcified plaques that are most prone to rupture. It also has a specific quirk in patients already on statin therapy: as Chapter 3 explained, statins may cause soft plaque to calcify and stabilize. This means that a rising calcium score in a treated patient may actually reflect plaque stabilization—a good thing—rather than deterioration. The CAC scan is best used to assess baseline cardiovascular risk in people who have not yet started treatment. It is generally not appropriate for low-risk patients, in whom a positive result generates anxiety and often leads to unnecessary invasive tests.

Stress Test

Contrary to common belief, routine stress tests are not part of an annual physical for healthy people without symptoms. A resting EKG can serve as a useful baseline and may reveal subtle electrical abnormalities, but a treadmill stress test is reserved for patients who have symptoms of possible heart disease—chest pain or tightness, unexplained shortness of breath during exertion, or significant cardiovascular risk with specific concerns. The stress test measures how effectively the heart responds to the increased demand of exercise. Nuclear stress tests, which use radioactive tracers, can map blood flow to different regions of the heart and identify areas that are not receiving enough blood flow during exertion.

Coronary Angiogram

When medications fail to control chest pain, or when a stress test raises significant concern, the next step is usually a coronary angiogram—a procedure in which a thin catheter is threaded into an artery at the wrist or groin, contrast dye is injected, and real-time X-ray images of the coronary arteries are captured. This remains the most direct way to visualize blockages and plan treatment. A newer, less invasive alternative—coronary CT angiography (CCTA)—has become the first-line tool to examine the coronary arteries without catheterization. A negative CCTA effectively rules out significant coronary disease, sparing the patient an invasive procedure. CCTA also provides information about both calcified and non-calcified plaque, giving a fuller picture of vulnerability than a CAC score alone. Coronary angiography is increasingly reserved for patients who are highly likely to need an immediate intervention like a stent.

Treatment of Coronary Artery Disease

Degree of Narrowing (Stenosis) of Heart Arteries Versus Outcomes

One of the most important conceptual shifts in cardiology over the past two decades is the recognition that the degree of narrowing in an artery—its stenosis percentage—is not the same thing as its functional importance. A blockage that looks severe on imaging may produce minimal restriction to blood flow, while a less dramatic narrowing in a critical location may be severely limiting. Current practice therefore prioritizes functional assessment: measuring the physiological significance of a blockage under conditions of maximal stress, not just its visual appearance. This shift has important practical implications. Some lesions with less than 70 percent stenosis may need treatment because they are causing symptoms that cannot be managed otherwise. Patients with even greater narrowing may be safely managed with medication alone if they are asymptomatic. Intervention is clearly indicated during an acute heart attack, or when there is more than 50 percent narrowing of the left main coronary artery—the dominant vessel supplying the bulk of the left heart muscle.

The standard functional assessment is fractional flow reserve (FFR) measurement: a wire with a pressure sensor is advanced past the blockage, and pressure is measured before and after the blockage under conditions of maximal blood flow. If the pressure drop across the blockage is significant, stent placement may be justified.

Stents

A stent is a small wire mesh tube placed inside a narrowed artery to prop it open and restore blood flow. During a heart attack, stenting is lifesaving: it opens the blocked vessel, stops the infarction in progress, preserves heart muscle, and dramatically reduces mortality. No question. But outside of the acute setting, the evidence tells a more complicated story. Experts estimate that roughly one in five stents is placed unnecessarily. This matters because stenting is not a trivial procedure—it carries real risks and may not improve outcomes. In patients with stable coronary artery disease—meaning chronic narrowing without an acute event—stenting can relieve chest pain that persists despite optimal medical therapy, enabling greater physical activity and improving quality of life. It is also preferred over bypass surgery when the left main artery is blocked, or when multiple critical blockages are anatomically suitable to stenting. Patients with refractory chest pain, heart failure, or high-risk stress test findings may be reasonable candidates for stenting. But here is the critical point: stents do not prevent future heart attacks in stable coronary disease, and they do not prolong life. Large, well-conducted randomized trials have shown that for stable CAD without ongoing symptoms, optimal medical therapy—aspirin, statins, blood pressure control, and lifestyle modification—produces equivalent outcomes to stenting. This is not a reason to avoid stenting when symptoms genuinely warrant it. It is a reason to consider a second opinion if you have no symptoms and your cardiologist is recommending a stent based on the appearance of your arteries alone.

Bypass Surgery

Coronary artery bypass graft surgery (CABG) is reserved for situations where stenting cannot do the job—most commonly when there are blockages in multiple major vessels, when the left main coronary artery is severely diseased, or when blockage anatomy makes stenting technically unsuitable. Patients with diabetes and multiple blockages tend to fare better with CABG than stenting, as do patients with significantly reduced heart function. In CABG surgery, a blood vessel harvested from the leg, arm, or chest wall is surgically rerouted around the blockage, creating a new conduit for blood flow. CABG is major surgery, with a six to twelve week recovery time, but for complex disease it offers durable, long-lasting results that stenting often cannot match. Both approaches—done for the right indications—reduce angina and improve activity tolerance. The key is matching the intervention to the anatomy and the patient.

Heart Failure

Heart failure affects about 1 in 100 people before age 50 and rises to roughly 1 in 10 among those over 80—a tenfold increase that reflects both the cumulative damage from decades of uncontrolled cardiovascular risk factors and the normal aging changes described at the start of this chapter. Heart failure is not the same as the heart "stopping"—it means the heart can no longer pump enough blood to meet the body's needs. The hallmark symptoms are shortness of breath, fatigue, and fluid retention (swollen ankles, weight gain from accumulated fluid). Diagnosis is based primarily on the ejection fraction (EF). In preserved EF heart failure (EF above 50 percent), the heart pumps normally but the muscle is stiff and does not fill properly. In reduced EF heart failure (EF below 40 percent), the heart muscle is weak and cannot generate adequate force.

Treatment for heart failure has expanded significantly. The foundation remains blood pressure medications (see Chapter 3)—ACE inhibitors or ARBs, beta blockers like metoprolol, and diuretics to clear excess fluid. A newer and remarkably effective addition is the SGLT2 inhibitor class (also called gliflozins): dapagliflozin (Farxiga), empagliflozin (Jardiance), and canagliflozin (Invokana) have all been shown to significantly reduce hospitalizations and deaths from heart failure, in patients with both preserved and reduced ejection fraction. These drugs were originally developed for diabetes, and their cardiac benefits came as a welcome surprise.

SGLT2 inhibitors work by blocking glucose reabsorption in the kidneys, causing excess sugar to be excreted in the urine. This produces modest weight loss (typically 5 to 6 pounds) and reductions in blood pressure, both of which help the failing heart. But the glucose in the urine also creates risks: dehydration, blood pressure drops, and an increased susceptibility to genital fungal infections and urinary tract infections. Because these drugs can trigger ketoacidosis, they are not used in patients with type 1 diabetes. We will explore their role in managing type 2 diabetes more fully in Chapter 7.

One more important addition to the heart failure arsenal: sacubitril/valsartan (Entresto), which combines an ARB (valsartan) with another drug to reduce cardiac stress in ways that standard ARBs alone cannot. It has shown particular benefit in female patients with reduced ejection fraction, and emerging evidence supports its use in heart failure with preserved EF as well. Like SGLT2 inhibitors, this drug decreases hospitalizations and deaths from heart failure, while also slowing decline of kidney function (see Chapters 7 and 15). This drug has shown an even stronger benefit in diabetics with heart failure and kidney disease.

Atrial Fibrillation

Atrial fibrillation (AF)—an irregular, often rapid quivering of the heart's upper chambers—affects more than 1 in 10 people over 65, making it the most common sustained heart rhythm disorder in older adults. In AF, the atria fire chaotically rather than contracting in an organized beat, reducing the heart's pumping efficiency and producing symptoms that range from a fluttering or racing sensation and lightheadedness to fatigue and breathlessness. Cardioversion—a controlled electrical shock to reset the heart's rhythm—is used immediately when AF produces dangerously low blood pressure, acute heart failure, or severe chest pain. For more stable patients who have been in AF for more than a week and are symptomatic, cardioversion may be attempted, though success rates are lower the longer the arrhythmia has been present.

The most dangerous consequence of atrial fibrillation is a stroke (see Chapter 5). When the atria quiver rather than contract, blood pools and can clot. If a clot travels to the brain, it can block an artery and cause a stroke. Preventing this is a primary goal of AF management. Long-term anticoagulation—blood thinning—is the standard approach. Newer anticoagulants (like apixaban and rivaroxaban) do not require regular blood monitoring and have a more predictable effect than older options. Warfarin (Coumadin) remains a cost-effective alternative but requires careful monitoring with regular blood tests. Before cardioversion, patients are typically anticoagulated for at least three weeks and an echocardiogram is usually performed to confirm no clots are present in the atria before attempting to restore rhythm.

Conclusion

Heart disease is the leading cause of death in the developed world—but its course is not fixed. Here is what this chapter asks you to remember. Chest discomfort, jaw or arm pain, shortness of breath, nausea, or unusual fatigue—especially in women, where symptoms are often atypical—are emergencies. The heart muscle begins dying within 20 to 30 minutes of a complete blockage. Every minute of delay means more irreversible damage. Time is muscle.

Call 911 immediately if you suspect a heart attack—and do not drive yourself. Next, chew four 81 mg baby aspirin or one regular (325 mg) aspirin which can limit the extent of heart muscle damage. If there is a suspicion of a stomach ulcer, GI bleed, symptoms of a stroke (see Chapter 5) or aspirin allergy, taking aspirin may be harmful.

For stable coronary artery disease without ongoing symptoms, optimal medical therapy—aspirin, statins, blood pressure control, and lifestyle modification—produces outcomes equivalent to stenting. Stents are lifesaving during a heart attack, but they do not prevent future attacks or extend life in stable disease.

Heart failure treatment has moved from just treating symptoms to actually slowing the disease, protecting the kidneys and living longer. SGLT2 inhibitors (dapagliflozin, empagliflozin) and sacubitril/valsartan (Entresto) have significantly reduced hospitalizations and deaths in both preserved and reduced ejection fraction heart failure, while also slowing kidney decline. For atrial fibrillation, the most dangerous consequence is stroke. Long-term anticoagulation—not aspirin—is the cornerstone of management.

Everything in this chapter connects back to the same upstream targets covered in Chapters 2 and 3: control your blood pressure (below 120 systolic), lower your LDL (below 70), do not smoke, and exercise regularly. The next chapter shows how these same risk factors damage the brain's blood vessels—and what you can do about it.

Chapter 5:

Blood Vessel Disease of the Brain

WHILE HEART DISEASE (CHAPTERS 3 and 4) is the first leading cause of death, stroke is the second leading cause and the leading cause of long-term disability worldwide. It is, in essence, a heart attack of the brain: the same process of atherosclerosis that narrows coronary arteries silently narrows the arteries supplying the brain—until a clot forms, a vessel ruptures, or blood flow simply stops. And just as every minute of delay during a heart attack costs irreplaceable heart muscle, every minute of delay during a stroke costs irreplaceable brain tissue. The numbers are stark: roughly 2 million brain cells die every minute a stroke goes untreated. "Time is brain" is not a slogan; it is the biology of the emergency.

How to Save Brain Tissue During a "Brain Attack"

Ischemic Stroke

About 90 percent of all strokes are ischemic: a brain artery becomes blocked, either by a clot that forms locally (thrombosis) or one that originates elsewhere in the body and travels to the brain (embolism). Atrial fibrillation—the irregular heart rhythm discussed in the previous chapter—is one of the most common causes of embolic stroke, which is why people with AF are prescribed anticoagulants. The remaining 10 percent of strokes are hemorrhagic, and these are covered in the next section.

Hemorrhagic Stroke

Hemorrhagic strokes are less common but often more immediately catastrophic. They occur when a blood vessel in or around the brain ruptures—either as an intracerebral hemorrhage (bleeding directly into the brain tissue) or a subarachnoid hemorrhage (bleeding into the fluid-filled space surrounding the brain). In both cases, the escaped blood rapidly forms a hematoma (blood clot) that expands, destroying nearby tissue and raising pressure inside the brain. Unlike ischemic strokes, clot-dissolving drugs are not just ineffective here—they are dangerous. The immediate priority is surgical: stop the bleeding, relieve the pressure, and prevent further damage.

Transient Ischemic Attack (TIA)

A transient ischemic attack (TIA)—commonly called a "mini-stroke"—is a stroke whose symptoms resolve completely within 24 hours, typically within minutes. The word "transient" is misleading: a TIA is not a minor event. It is the most urgent warning the brain can send. Without proper treatment, the risk of a full stroke after a TIA is as high as 15 percent within the first 90 days, and nearly half of those strokes occur within 48 hours of the TIA. A TIA must be treated as the same emergency as a full stroke. Call 911. Do not wait to see if symptoms return. The window for prevention is measured in hours, not days.

"Brain Attack" Treatment: This Could Save Your Life!

Treatment for stroke is time-critical in a way that few other medical emergencies match. For ischemic stroke, the goal is to restore blood flow before brain tissue dies. Arriving at a certified stroke center within 3 to 4.5 hours of symptom onset makes patients eligible for intravenous thrombolysis—a clot-dissolving drug that can dramatically limit damage. For larger vessel blockages, mechanical thrombectomy—a catheter-based procedure that physically retrieves the clot—can be performed up to 24 hours after onset in carefully selected patients, with outcomes that were unimaginable a decade ago. For hemorrhagic stroke, speed is even more critical: emergency surgery to evacuate the blood, clip the ruptured vessel, or place a shunt to relieve intracranial pressure may be the only chance to prevent death or severe disability. Every hospital is not equally equipped—getting to a certified stroke center, not just the nearest emergency room, can be the difference between full recovery and permanent disability. If you cannot get to a stroke center, a local emergency room will do a brain CT to rule out a bleed; if there is no bleed, they will give the clot-busting drug. Once this is done and a patient is stable, they are moved to a certified stroke center.

Stroke Symptoms: BEFAST— A Method to Save Lives

Knowing the warning signs of stroke is one of the highest-value things you can do for the people around you. Most strokes happen in the presence of a bystander—a family member, a colleague, a friend—who has the power to call 911 before irreversible damage is done. The acronym FASTBE captures the most important signs to watch for. Every letter is a potential lifesaver:

- "F" — Face: Ask the person to smile. Does one side of their face droop?
- "A" — Arms: Ask them to raise both arms. Does one arm drift downward?
- "S" — Speech: Ask them to repeat a simple sentence. Are their words slurred? Can they say it correctly?
- "T" — Time: Note when the first symptoms appeared, as this information is essential for healthcare providers.
- "B" — Balance: Sudden loss of balance, dizziness, or difficulty walking.
- "E" — Eyes: Blurred vision, double vision, or loss of vision.

T for Time the most critical letter in FASTBE—noting when symptoms first appeared tells the treatment team exactly how long the brain has been deprived of blood, which determines which treatments are still possible. Beyond the FASTBE signs, watch for sudden numbness or weakness on one side of the body, sudden severe headache with no obvious cause (often described as "the worst headache of my life"), sudden confusion, or difficulty understanding what others are saying. If any of these appear: call 911 immediately, note the time, and ask for transport to a certified stroke center. Do not drive the person yourself—paramedics can begin evaluation and treatment in the ambulance, before you arrive at the hospital.

Atherosclerosis of the Small Blood Vessels in the Brain

Not all strokes announce themselves dramatically. Small vessel disease—the narrowing or blockage of the brain's tiny penetrating arteries—can produce "silent" strokes, called lacunar infarcts, that cause no obvious symptoms at the time they occur. Over months and years, however, the damage adds up. Symptoms of small vessel disease depend on which brain regions are affected, and may include subtle weakness or numbness on one side of the body, difficulty finding words, balance problems, shuffling steps, and an increased risk of falls. Cognitively, the damage may begin as attention difficulties and forgetfulness before progressing to vascular dementia—a form of cognitive decline driven directly by accumulated vascular injury. Small vessel disease follows the same pattern as large vessel atherosclerosis: years of uncontrolled blood pressure and high LDL, causing cumulative damage that eventually becomes irreversible. The interventions that prevent it are identical: control blood pressure, control cholesterol, do not smoke, exercise, and eat well.

Treatment Options to Reduce Stroke Risk

Stroke prevention is largely the same as heart attack prevention—because the underlying disease is the same. Controlling blood pressure is the single most powerful intervention: hypertension is the dominant modifiable risk factor for both ischemic and hemorrhagic stroke. Lowering LDL with statins reduces ischemic stroke risk substantially. Not smoking, exercising regularly, and eating a Mediterranean-style diet all contribute. For patients who have already had a TIA or ischemic stroke, low-dose aspirin significantly reduces the risk of recurrence unless bleeding risk is high or atrial fibrillation is present (in which case anticoagulation is preferred). A newer and notable development: GLP-1 receptor agonists, originally developed for type 2 diabetes, have been shown in clinical trials to reduce ischemic stroke risk—enough that both the American Heart Association and the American Stroke Association now recommend considering them for primary stroke prevention in patients with diabetes and elevated cardiovascular risk. For patients with atrial fibrillation, anticoagulation—not aspirin—is the cornerstone of stroke prevention, and anticoagulation should not be delayed or substituted.

Conclusion

Stroke is a brain attack, and it deserves the same urgency we have learned to give a heart attack. The biology is unforgiving—2 million brain cells per minute, lost permanently—but the window for intervention is real, and what happens in the first hour after symptom onset often determines the rest of a person's life. Know FASTBE. Know that a TIA is an emergency, not a near-miss to monitor at home. Know that the goal is a certified stroke center, not just the nearest hospital. Prevention of strokes can be aided by not smoking, eating a healthy diet and meeting blood pressure, LDL cholesterol and exercise goals described in prior chapters. In the next chapter we will review things to maintain your brain function into old age, which includes slowing atherosclerosis of brain blood vessels.

Chapter 6:

How to Maintain Brain and Nervous System Function into Old Age

THE FEAR OF LOSING one's cognitive function is, for many people, more frightening than the fear of death. Research suggests that up to 45 percent of dementia cases could be prevented or meaningfully delayed through lifestyle interventions. This chapter explains which interventions work, and how to put them into practice. At the center of it all is a concept called neuroplasticity—the brain's remarkable capacity to adapt, reorganize, and even grow throughout life.

Age and Its Effects on the Brain and Nervous System

The brain is the most complex structure in the known universe: roughly 86 billion neurons, each connected to up to 10,000 others, forming approximately 100 trillion connections. This network is the physical substrate of everything you think, feel, remember, and do. With age, some of that complexity naturally diminishes. Nerve cells are lost. Connections between them weaken. The brain's volume gradually shrinks. Processing speed slows—you notice that it takes a moment longer to retrieve a name, to shift between tasks, to react. Levels of important chemicals involved in communication between nerve cells may decrease, affecting mood, motivation and emotions (see Chapter 18), but the brain has this remarkable ability to adapt.

How to Slow Age-Related Brain Changes: Neuroplasticity

The most important thing neuroscience has taught us in the past three decades is that the brain never stops adapting. Neuroplasticity—the brain's ability to reorganize its structure, forge new connections, strengthen existing ones, and even generate new nerve cells (neurons)—persists throughout life, well into old age. After a stroke, for instance, the brain can reroute functions from damaged areas to intact regions—a process that physical therapy helps accelerate. At the molecular level, a protein called Brain-Derived Neurotrophic Factor (BDNF) does much of this work. BDNF acts as fertilizer for the brain: it promotes the growth of new neurons, strengthens connections between nerve cells, which supports learning, memory, and higher-level thinking. BDNF levels are not fixed by genetics. They rise with exercise, mental stimulation, and good sleep, and they fall with chronic stress, social isolation, and sedentary behavior. The practical implication is enormous: the choices you make every day are shaping the physical architecture of your brain.

The brain, like a muscle, responds to challenge—and that challenge does not have to come from your job. Mentally engaging activities pursued at any point in life—puzzles, learning a new instrument, studying a language, reading deeply, playing strategy games—stimulate BDNF production and build what researchers call cognitive reserve: a buffer of extra neural capacity that allows the brain to maintain function even as it sustains damage. People with higher cognitive reserve show fewer symptoms of Alzheimer's at equivalent levels of brain tissue damage. The brain can be carrying considerable disease while still functioning well, because it has more to draw on. What you do in your leisure hours matters just as much as what you do at work—perhaps more, since you control it entirely. Lifelong learning is not merely enriching—it is protective. Take it seriously as a health practice.

Exercise and Your Brain

If there is a single intervention with the strongest evidence for protecting the aging brain, it is exercise. Exercise increases blood flow to the brain, triggers robust BDNF production, promotes neurogenesis (the formation of new neurons) in the hippocampus—the brain's primary memory center—and reduces the chronic inflammation that accelerates deterioration of the nervous system. Regular aerobic exercise is associated with meaningfully lower rates of Alzheimer's and other forms of dementia. The prescription is the same as for heart health: at least 150 minutes of moderate aerobic activity per week (walking, jogging, cycling, swimming), plus resistance training at least twice a week. The brain and heart respond to the same medicine.

Your Social Network

Social connection is, neurologically, a form of exercise for the brain. Conversation, emotional engagement, the give-and-take of relationships—these are cognitively demanding activities that stimulate neural networks and support BDNF production. The research is unambiguous: older adults with active social lives have substantially lower rates of dementia than those who are socially isolated (see Chapter 18). Loneliness is not merely unpleasant—it is a stressor that suppresses immune function, and accelerates cognitive decline. One longitudinal study found that individuals with a positive attitude toward aging lived an average of seven years longer than those with negative expectations. Your mindset about growing older, and your investment in relationships, are not soft lifestyle choices. They are medical ones.

Healthy Heart, Healthy Blood Vessels, Healthy Brain

The brain is supplied by many blood vessels, and what damages blood vessels damages the brain. Every cardiovascular risk factor—uncontrolled high blood pressure, high LDL cholesterol, type 2 diabetes, obesity, smoking—is simultaneously a risk factor for cognitive decline. Atherosclerosis of the brain's small vessels can cause silent lacunar infarcts (see Chapter 5), which can lead to vascular dementia. Smoking specifically has been linked to accelerated brain atrophy, cognitive decline, and a substantially elevated stroke risk. The most powerful things you can do for your brain—controlling blood pressure to below 120 systolic, keeping LDL below 70, exercising, eating a Mediterranean diet, and not smoking—are the same things covered in Chapters 1 through 5. Brain health and cardiovascular health are not separate projects.

Your Diet and Your Brain

Food choice can significantly impact brain health. The

Mediterranean diet—abundant in vegetables, fruits, whole grains, legumes, fatty fish, nuts, and olive oil—is associated with meaningfully slower cognitive decline and reduced Alzheimer's risk, driven by its high concentrations of antioxidants and anti-inflammatory omega-3 fatty acids. At the other end of the spectrum, ultra-processed foods and high-sugar diets drive chronic systemic inflammation—a process that accelerates decline of the nervous system (neurodegeneration). Large epidemiological studies have found that people who consume the most ultra-processed foods show significantly faster rates of cognitive decline than those who consume the least. The brain's immune cells (microglia) are like first responders that keep the brain healthy. But when overstimulated, they can contribute to neurodegeneration. High saturated fats and high-sugar diets push the microglia into overdrive, while omega-3 fatty acids can turn down the inflammatory response (see Chapter 16).

Supplements and Your Brain

The supplement industry has generated enormous interest in products that claim to protect the aging brain—and an equally enormous amount of misleading evidence to support them. For healthy individuals who eat a reasonably varied diet, the consistent finding across large, well-designed trials is that supplements—multivitamins, individual vitamins C and E, beta-carotene, most herbal preparations—do not reduce rates of cognitive decline, cancer, heart disease, or mortality. Unlike prescription medications, dietary supplements are not approved by the FDA for safety or efficacy, may contain contaminants including heavy metals and pesticides, and can interact with medications in ways that reduce effectiveness or cause harm.

There are genuine exceptions—specific deficiencies in specific populations. People following strict vegan or paleo diets with severe dairy restrictions may be deficient in vitamin B12, calcium, or vitamin D, and supplementation is appropriate in those cases. The key word is deficiency: supplementing when you are not deficient adds nothing.

High-dose fish oil supplements (over 3 grams per day) carry an increased risk of developing atrial fibrillation. By contrast, getting omega-3 fatty acids from your diet—fatty fish, walnuts, flaxseed—is associated with a lower risk of atrial fibrillation. If you do want to take fish oil, there is some evidence that doses up to 3 grams per day may slow memory loss in patients with mild cognitive impairment.

Vitamin D deficiency is associated with increased cognitive decline risk, and supplementation is reasonable if blood levels are low and dietary and sun exposure are insufficient—but do not exceed 4,000 IU per day without medical guidance. In one study of patients who were not clinically deficient in vitamin D, supplemental vitamin D was associated with accelerated decline in mental function. Ginkgo biloba, despite decades of marketing for memory, has consistently failed to demonstrate meaningful benefit in rigorous trials. Vitamin E, curcumin, and CoQ10 share the same problem: compelling lab data, disappointing results in humans at scale. Unless future evidence supports these brain supplements, my advice is: get all the nutrients you need from a Mediterranean-type diet.

Alcohol and Your Brain

Alcohol can be toxic to the brain. Moderate to heavy drinking—a threshold much lower than most people assume—accelerates cognitive decline, shrinks brain volume, impairs neuroplasticity, and significantly increases the risk of early-onset dementia. The mechanisms are direct: alcohol damages neurons, disrupts the blood-brain barrier, and suppresses BDNF production. It also disrupts sleep architecture (even when it seems to help you fall asleep), worsens anxiety and depression, and compounds other dementia risk factors. For brain health, the evidence increasingly supports limiting alcohol consumption significantly—or eliminating it.

Caffeine

Caffeine deserves its reputation as a cognitive enhancer—at least in moderation. Caffeine can sharpen alertness, focus, and reaction time, and the evidence for its long-term benefits is encouraging. Multiple large studies have found associations between moderate coffee consumption (roughly 3 to 5 cups per day) and reduced risk of both Alzheimer's and Parkinson's disease—a finding that has held up across different populations and study methods. The mechanism is not fully established, but caffeine's anti-inflammatory properties and its effects on brain receptors are likely involved. The caveat: excessive intake produces anxiety, disturbs sleep (which itself damages the brain), and can impair the cognitive function it is meant to support. Moderate and consistent is the approach that works.

Sleep and Mental Function

Sleep is not passive. During deep sleep, the brain activates a waste-clearance system called the glymphatic system, which flushes out metabolic byproducts—including the amyloid plaques and tau tangles associated with Alzheimer's disease. Chronically poor sleep allows these waste products to accumulate. BDNF production drops. Memory consolidation—the process by which the day's experiences are encoded into long-term memory—is impaired. Immune function weakens. The risk of type 2 diabetes, obesity, heart disease, and stroke all rise. Sleep disorders like sleep apnea, which are common in older adults and often undiagnosed, are independently associated with accelerated cognitive decline. Recent research has added another dimension: it is not just sleep duration that matters, but sleep regularity. A consistent sleep schedule—going to bed and waking at roughly the same time each day—predicts long-term health outcomes more powerfully than any particular sleep duration, possibly because it preserves the brain's circadian rhythms, which govern everything from hormone production to emotional regulation.

Managing Insomnia

Treating insomnia begins with behavior, not pills. The most effective non-pharmacological treatment is Cognitive Behavioral Therapy (CBT) for Insomnia, which addresses the thought patterns and habits that perpetuate sleeplessness—and produces more durable results than any medication. The practical toolkit: maintain a consistent sleep and wake time seven days a week; keep the bedroom cool (60–67°F / 15–19°C), dark, and reserved for sleep; limit caffeine after midday and alcohol entirely near bedtime; avoid vigorous exercise in the two hours before sleep; and cut screen exposure at least an hour before bed, since blue-spectrum light suppresses melatonin. A weighted blanket and quality bedding are small investments that many people find genuinely helpful.

Buddhist Meditation Music for Sleep

I want to share something personal here. I have struggled with insomnia for most of my adult life, and I have tried most of the standard interventions. The combination that has worked best for me is simple: a hot bath, cold dark bedroom, a good supportive memory foam mattress and pillow, a weighted type blanket and Buddhist meditation music—specifically the resonant tones of Tibetan singing bowls and gongs. The sounds are rhythmic and non-verbal, which gives the mind something to follow without demanding the kind of active engagement that keeps us awake. Over time, the brain begins to associate these sounds with sleep, creating a conditioned "sleep trigger." I offer this as an example of how effective non-pharmacological tools can be when you find the ones that work for you.

Medications for Insomnia

When behavioral strategies are not enough, medications can help—but the hierarchy matters. Melatonin (0.5 to 5 mg taken 30 to 60 minutes before bed) is a reasonable first option for circadian rhythm disruption and jet lag. On the downside, a recent study found an association between long-term melatonin use and increased risk of heart failure hospitalizations; other studies suggest any benefit is quite small. Over-the-counter antihistamines like diphenhydramine (Benadryl) are widely used but poorly suited for the aging brain: they cause daytime grogginess, impair cognition, and are associated with increased dementia risk with long-term use—a serious concern. Prescription sedative-hypnotics like zolpidem (Ambien) and eszopiclone (Lunesta) are effective for short-term use but carry real risks in older adults: falls, fractures, next-day impairment, and tolerance (the need for progressively higher doses) that typically develops within three months. These sedative-hypnotic drugs are intended for short-term use with close follow-up. A better prescription option for many patients are low-dose antidepressants used off-label for insomnia—trazodone in particular—which improve sleep quality with lower dependence risk, though side effects like dry mouth and constipation warrant attention. Whatever medication is considered, the goal should be the minimum effective dose for the shortest necessary period, while working toward behavioral solutions that last. Always consult with your health care provider before resorting to sleep-inducing medications.

Power Nap

For older adults like myself, I enjoy my afternoon "power nap." Studies show that a simple rest period of 20 to 40 minutes may improve cognitive function and may slow brain aging. While a short nap is restorative, excessive daytime napping is viewed as a potential early warning sign of neurodegeneration—

loss of functional brain tissue. In the early stages of Alzheimer's, patients often take longer daytime naps, and napping for over one hour is associated with faster future cognitive decline. The most effective time for a nap is during the post-lunch dip in alertness between 1 PM and 3 PM. Napping after 4 PM can make it harder to fall asleep at night. If you find that a 20-minute nap leaves you feeling refreshed and your nighttime sleep remains solid, it is likely one of the best "free" longevity tools at your disposal. However, if you find yourself needing more than an hour of sleep every afternoon just to function, it may be worth discussing with your physician to rule out sleep apnea or early-stage changes in brain health.

Reduce Stress to Help Your Brain

Chronic stress is corrosive to the brain in ways that are now well understood. Persistently elevated cortisol—the primary stress hormone—suppresses BDNF production, damages neurons in the hippocampus (the memory center), impairs decision-making, and accelerates cognitive decline. Stress can actually lead to remodeling of brain structure over time. The antidotes are also well-established. Mindfulness meditation, yoga, deep breathing exercises, regular physical activity, and CBT all reduce cortisol, raise BDNF, and improve cognitive outcomes. The challenge is consistency—these practices work the way exercise works: reliably and cumulatively, but only if you do them. One simple technique to reduce stress that does not require any devices or medications is to practice slow breathing. You might want to try the 4-7-8 calm breathing exercise video on YouTube.

Preventing Cognitive Decline From Alzheimer's and Parkinson's Disease

The headline finding from decades of dementia research is both humbling and empowering: up to 40 percent of Alzheimer's and other dementia cases are estimated to be preventable or delayable through lifestyle change. The risk factors are the same ones covered throughout this book—high blood pressure (the single strongest modifiable risk factor for dementia), type 2 diabetes, obesity, physical inactivity, smoking, social isolation, depression, hearing loss, and traumatic brain injury. For Parkinson's specifically, balance and gait-focused activities like Tai Chi and yoga, and aerobic exercise including cycling, have shown promising effects on both motor and cognitive decline. Hearing loss deserves special mention: it forces the brain to devote extra cognitive resources to processing sound, leaving fewer for memory and thinking. Treating hearing loss with hearing aids appears to meaningfully reduce dementia risk—one of the more cost-effective interventions available. Protect your head: traumatic brain injury is a known trigger for both Parkinson's and Alzheimer's, and helmets for cycling and fall-prevention strategies (see Chapter 10) for older adults are not optional precautions. They are evidence-based medicine.

Shingles Vaccine and Dementia

An unexpected finding has emerged from recent research:

vaccination against shingles (herpes zoster) appears to be associated with a reduced risk of dementia—including Alzheimer's—as well as lower rates of heart attack and stroke. The mechanism is not yet fully understood, and more research is needed to confirm the relationship. What is already established is that shingles itself is a serious and painful condition: the nerve pain it causes (postherpetic neuralgia) can be severe and last for months or years. The two-dose shingles vaccine produces a few days of flu-like symptoms that most people find genuinely unpleasant—but given the severity of the disease it prevents, and the emerging evidence of additional benefits, the temporary discomfort is a worthwhile trade-off.

Conclusion

The central message of this chapter is one of genuine optimism: the brain is not a fixed machine that runs down as you age. It is a living, adaptive system—shaped by neuroplasticity throughout life—that responds powerfully to how you treat it. Up to 45 percent of dementia cases are estimated to be preventable through choices that are largely in your hands.

Regular aerobic exercise is the single strongest evidence-based intervention for brain health at any age. A Mediterranean-style eating pattern protects the brain through anti-inflammatory omega-3 fatty acids and antioxidants, while ultra-processed foods accelerate the inflammation that hastens cognitive decline. Controlling blood pressure below 120 systolic and LDL below 70 is as important for your brain as it is for your heart—because what damages blood vessels damages the brain.

Not smoking, and sharply limiting alcohol will also help to maintain brain health.

Getting good sleep, minimizing stress and maximizing social connections are biologic necessities for brain health.

None of this requires perfection, and none of it requires a demanding job or a privileged lifestyle. A daily walk. A Mediterranean meal. A good night's sleep. A phone call with a friend. An hour with a book or a puzzle. These are some of the building blocks of a brain that ages well.

Chapter 7:

How to Reverse Diabetes and Reduce Its Harmful Effects

DIABETES IS ONE OF the most consequential diagnoses in modern medicine—not primarily because of what high blood sugar does on its own, but because of what it does to every blood vessel in the body. Diabetes accelerates atherosclerosis, damages the tiny vessels supplying the eyes, kidneys, and nerves, and dramatically raises the risk of heart attack, stroke, heart failure, and kidney failure. It may also, in some cases, be reversible. This chapter examines what diabetes is, how it is diagnosed, what its complications look like, and—most importantly—how lifestyle changes and a new generation of medications now make it possible not just to manage type 2 diabetes, but to put it into remission.

Diabetes Types and Prevalence

Diabetes affects more than one in ten adults worldwide—and in the United States, approximately one in three people over 65 carries the diagnosis. The vast majority have type 2 diabetes, a condition in which the body produces insulin but cannot use it effectively, a problem called insulin resistance. Type 1 diabetes is fundamentally different: it is an auto-immune disease (where the body's protective system turns on itself) in which the pancreas produces no insulin at all, requiring lifelong insulin replacement. Some patients with long-standing type 2 diabetes eventually need insulin, as the pancreas's capacity to produce it diminishes over time.

Diabetes Diagnosis / Symptoms

Type 2 diabetes is diagnosed through two measurements: fasting blood glucose and hemoglobin A1C (HbA1c), which reflects the average blood sugar level over the preceding two to three months. Normal is a fasting glucose below 100 mg/dL and an A1C below 5.7 percent. Prediabetes—the warning zone that often precedes full diabetes—is defined as a fasting glucose of 100 to 125 mg/dL or an A1C of 5.7 to 6.4 percent. Diabetes is diagnosed at a fasting glucose at or above 125 mg/dL and 126 mg/dL or an A1C at or above 6.5 percent. Typical symptoms include increased thirst, frequent urination, unusual hunger, blurred vision, fatigue, and wounds that heal slowly. If you have any of these, have your blood sugar tested.

Diabetes Complications

Even prediabetes carries meaningful risks. The long-term damage to the heart, blood vessels and kidneys may begin in the prediabetic stage. Prediabetics are nearly twice as likely to have a heart attack and are at a higher risk of strokes and heart failure compared to patients with normal blood glucose levels. That risk increases dramatically with full type 2 diabetes, where the likelihood of heart attack, stroke, and heart failure is 2 to 4 times higher than in non-diabetics.

The risk of complications correlates directly with how high blood sugar rises and for how long it stays elevated—which is why early intervention matters. But the picture has grown more nuanced: controlling blood sugar alone is no longer the primary goal of modern diabetes treatment.

Reaching target blood pressure and LDL cholesterol levels is, for diabetic patients, at least as important as controlling blood sugar. Adding SGLT2 inhibitors and GLP-1 receptor agonists—drugs that do more than lower glucose—has been shown to reduce heart attacks, stroke, heart failure, and kidney failure in diabetic patients independently of their effects on blood sugar. This is a fundamental shift in how we think about the disease.

Prevention of Small Vessel Disease Complications

The damage diabetes does to small blood vessels can lead to diabetic eye, kidney and nerve complications. After decades of elevated glucose, roughly half of all people with type 1 diabetes and one-third of those with type 2 develop one or more of three classic small vessel complications. Diabetic retinopathy attacks the blood vessels of the retina; early detection through regular eye exams and, when needed, laser therapy can prevent the vision loss that retinopathy would otherwise cause. Diabetic neuropathy damages the nerves, typically starting in the feet and hands, producing numbness, tingling, and eventually severe pain; treatment options remain limited. Diabetic nephropathy damages the kidneys' filtering units, potentially progressing to kidney failure requiring dialysis. Even prediabetics carry a 10 to 15 percent elevated risk of all three conditions compared to people with normal blood sugar.

The clearest evidence we have for preventing small vessel complications comes from younger patients early in their disease: maintaining blood sugar close to normal from the beginning of the diabetes diagnosis significantly reduces the risk of retinopathy, neuropathy, and nephropathy. The earlier and more consistently this is done, the greater the benefit.

I have a close friend who has had type 1 diabetes since age 5. He has been very good about controlling his blood sugar levels, which has paid off by keeping him from developing diabetic eye and kidney disease.

A Non-Glucose Focused Approach to Diabetes Treatment

One of the most important conceptual shifts in diabetes medicine over the past decade is this: type 2 diabetes is no longer treated primarily as a disease of blood sugar. It is now understood as a complex, systemic disease driven largely by obesity and insulin resistance, whose most deadly manifestations are heart attacks, strokes and kidney failure. Modern treatment has reorganized its priorities. Rather than asking "how do we lower A1C," the first question is now "how do we protect the heart, brain, and kidneys—and how do we address the underlying obesity?" Blood sugar control remains important, but it has been moved to second position. The drugs that have earned first-line status—SGLT2 inhibitors and GLP-1 receptor agonists—were chosen not because they are the most potent glucose-lowering agents, but because they are the only diabetes drugs proven to reduce cardiovascular and kidney complications, extend life, and promote meaningful weight loss simultaneously. This "complications-first" philosophy is a genuine paradigm shift, and patients deserve to know about it.

Prevention of Large Vessel Disease Complications

Approximately two-thirds of deaths in diabetic patients are caused by atherosclerosis of large blood vessels—heart attacks, strokes, and peripheral artery disease—as described in Chapters 3 and 4. The relationship between glucose control and large vessel disease, however, is more complicated than it is for small vessel disease. Early tight glucose control in younger patients with type 1 or type 2 diabetes—before significant atherosclerosis has developed—appears to reduce future cardiovascular events, a benefit that persists for years after the period of tight control (called the "legacy effect"). But for patients with long-standing type 2 diabetes who already have established atherosclerosis, several large randomized trials found that aggressive glucose lowering was not beneficial and, in some cases, caused harm—particularly from dangerously low blood sugars (hypoglycemia). Thus the timing of blood sugar control matters as much as blood sugar targets.

Insulin is an essential therapy when oral medications cannot achieve adequate control—but it should not be the default. Insulin promotes weight gain, offers none of the cardiovascular or kidney-protective benefits of GLP-1 and SGLT2 drugs, requires injections and frequent glucose monitoring, and carries a real risk of hypoglycemia that is especially dangerous in older adults. When insulin is needed, it should be added thoughtfully and in the lowest effective dose.

SGLT-2 Drugs to Prevent Complications of Diabetes

SGLT2 inhibitors—dapagliflozin (Farxiga), empagliflozin (Jardiance), and canagliflozin (Invokana)—represent the most significant advance in diabetes treatment since insulin. Originally approved as glucose-lowering agents, they have proven to do far more. In patients with type 2 diabetes and established cardiovascular disease, SGLT2 inhibitors reduce the risk of major adverse cardiac events (heart attack, stroke, and cardiovascular death) by 14 percent and hospitalization for heart failure by more than 30 percent—benefits that are only partially explained by their modest glucose-lowering effect. The protective mechanism is unclear but may include a lower blood pressure, modest weight loss (typically 4 to 6 pounds), and direct effects on heart muscle cells. The kidney-protective effects are equally striking. SGLT2 inhibitors slow the progression of diabetic kidney disease across a wide range of kidney function. This means that a diabetic patient with heart failure and chronic kidney disease—a common combination—gets multiple benefits from a single drug class. For that reason, current guidelines from the American Diabetes Association, the American College of Cardiology, and the American Heart Association all recommend SGLT2 inhibitors as a first-line treatment whenever a diabetic patient has heart failure, chronic kidney disease, or established atherosclerotic cardiovascular disease (see Chapters 3 and 4), regardless of A1C levels.The benefits of SGLT2 inhibitors and their role in managing both heart failure and kidney disease are discussed further in Chapters 4 and 15.

A1C Targets and Age

Age-adjusted A1C targets are one of the most practically important concepts in diabetes management—and one of the least appreciated. The harm from aggressive glucose control in older patients comes primarily from hypoglycemia that can cause confusion, loss of consciousness, falls, and cardiac events. Older adults are more vulnerable to hypoglycemia than younger patients (their warning signs are often blunted or absent), and they have fewer years of glucose exposure ahead of them, meaning less time to benefit from tight control. For younger, newly diagnosed patients, an A1C target below 6.5 percent is appropriate and achievable. For older adults over 65—particularly those with established cardiovascular disease or kidney disease—a target of 7.5 to 8 percent is safer and more realistic. Adults over 65 have a nearly fourfold higher risk of hospitalization from hypoglycemia compared to younger patients. Treating an 80-year-old with the same intensity as a 45-year-old is not better medicine—it is a common and preventable cause of harm.

Reversing Diabetes: Lifestyle Issues

The possibility of putting type 2 diabetes into remission through diet and lifestyle is not a fringe idea—it is a well-documented clinical reality. The key lever is weight loss. Studies show that losing 10 to 15 percent of body weight lowers A1C, improves insulin sensitivity, and induces remission in 40 to 50 percent of cases. The dietary approach matters too. A very low-carbohydrate ketogenic diet (20 to 30 grams of carbs per day) can produce remission rates of around 50 percent, but it is difficult to sustain long-term and can cause nutritional deficiencies. I recommend a low-carbohydrate Mediterranean-style diet instead—approximately 40 percent of calories from carbohydrates—which achieves meaningful glucose improvement, supports heart health, and is far easier to maintain for years without counting every gram of glucose.

For people with prediabetes, the evidence for lifestyle intervention is particularly compelling. The landmark 2001 Diabetes Prevention Program trial showed that 150 minutes of physical activity weekly along with a low-carb diet, which led to weight loss, reduced the risk of developing diabetes by 58 percent compared to the control group. Other studies indicate that a weight loss of 10 to 15 percent—not unusual with GLP-1 weight loss drugs—can lower hemoglobin A1c, improve blood glucose levels and insulin sensitivity, and induce remission in a significant percentage of patients with type 2 diabetes.

Reversing Diabetes: Medications

GLP-1 receptor agonists (discussed in detail in Chapter 2) are now the most powerful pharmacological tool for achieving diabetes remission. They produce 10 to 15 percent body weight loss in diabetic patients, and combining them with lifestyle changes can double the remission rate compared to lifestyle alone. The catch: if the medication is stopped, elevated weight and blood sugar levels typically return. These are not one-time treatments—they are long-term therapies that work best when sustained.

Metformin remains a reasonable and inexpensive first medication for many patients, particularly when cost is a primary concern. It does not produce the dramatic weight loss or cardiovascular protection of SGLT2 and GLP-1 agents, but it is safe, well-tolerated, and has evidence supporting its role in slowing the progression from prediabetes to diabetes when combined with lifestyle measures. Like bariatric surgery, GLP-1 drugs improve the body's insulin response to meals—one reason both approaches can achieve remission beyond what caloric restriction alone would predict.

Bariatric Surgery to Reverse Diabetes

For patients with significant obesity who cannot achieve remission through diet, exercise, and medications alone, bariatric surgery remains the most powerful intervention available. Nearly all patients with prediabetes see normalization of blood sugar after bariatric surgery. More than half of those with established type 2 diabetes experience full remission. The surgery works partly through dramatic caloric restriction and partly through improved insulin sensitivity independent of weight loss. It is major surgery with real risks, but for the right patient, it can be genuinely curative.

Can Diabetes Remission Prevent Complications?

The most important unanswered question in diabetes medicine is whether achieving remission—whether through lifestyle, medication, or surgery—translates into prevention of long-term complications. Preliminary data are encouraging: remission appears to reduce small vessel disease complications and cardiovascular benefits have been observed in patients who lose substantial weight through bariatric surgery. But definitive long-term data on remission and complication prevention are still emerging.

Conclusion

Type 2 diabetes is one of the most consequential conditions in medicine. Its complications—heart attack, stroke, blindness, kidney failure, limb amputation—are among the most devastating outcomes in aging. But they are not inevitable. The modern approach to diabetes treatment has shifted from simply managing blood sugar to aggressively protecting the organs diabetes damages most: the heart, brain, and kidneys. SGLT2 inhibitors and GLP-1 receptor agonists do this better than any prior medications. Lifestyle change—particularly weight loss and exercise—can induce remission in a meaningful proportion of patients. Younger patients should pursue tight glucose control to protect against small vessel disease. Older patients should be managed with more conservative targets, prioritizing safety over numbers. Remember, remission is not a cure, it is a maintained state that requires continued effort and diabetes will return if lifestyle and diet are not sustained.

Long term studies are required to see if reversing type 2 diabetes will result in the slowing or prevention of the complications of diabetes.

Chapter 8:

Genes Are Not Destiny

MANY PEOPLE BELIEVE THAT their health destiny is written in their DNA—that if heart disease, Alzheimer's, or cancer runs in the family, it will affect them too. The science tells a more hopeful story. While genes provide the underlying blueprint, they are not the final word. The field of epigenetics has revealed that our lifestyle choices continuously modify how our genes behave—turning some on, silencing others, altering their effects in ways that compound over a lifetime. Communities around the world where people routinely live into their 90s and beyond share not a unique genetic endowment, but a common set of habits: plant-heavy diets, daily movement, strong social bonds, a sense of purpose. Their longevity appears to be, in large measure, earned. This chapter explains how genes work, how epigenetics modifies them, and why lifestyle choices discussed in prior chapters matter at the level of your DNA.

DNA, Chromosomes, and Genes

Genetics begins with chromosomes: 23 pairs of them in every human cell, one set inherited from each parent. Chromosomes are tightly coiled structures made of DNA (deoxyribonucleic acid) wrapped around proteins. Embedded within each chromosome are genes—specific sequences of DNA that serve as instructions for building proteins, the molecular machines that carry out virtually every function in the body.

DNA is built from four chemical letters—adenine (A), cytosine (C), guanine (G), and thymine (T)—arranged in billions of sequences that make up the human genome. These sequences encode instructions for manufacturing proteins from chains of amino acids. Your body cannot synthesize all the amino acids it needs on its own; the essential ones must come from protein-rich foods—meat, fish, eggs, dairy, beans, nuts, and seeds. When a gene is read, the cell's machinery assembles the corresponding protein according to its amino acid sequence—and that protein then goes to work, whether as an enzyme, a structural component, a hormone, or a signal molecule.

The intermediate step between DNA (the master blueprint) and protein (the finished product) is RNA (ribonucleic acid). RNA is a single-stranded molecule that copies a gene's instructions from DNA and carries them to ribosomes—the cell's protein factories—where amino acids are assembled in the correct sequence. The genetic code dictates how cells translate information from DNA and RNA into amino acid sequences that form proteins. Understanding this chain helps explain both how genes cause disease and how gene therapies aim to interrupt or correct that chain.

Which Genes Are Active?

Every cell in your body contains the same complete genome—roughly 20,000 genes. Yet a nerve cell looks and behaves nothing like a liver cell or a muscle cell. The reason is gene expression: only a subset of genes is active in any given cell type, and which genes are active determines what the cell does. This selective activation is controlled by regulatory regions of DNA—which account for the vast majority of the genome. Only about 1 to 2 percent of human DNA encodes actual proteins; the remaining 98 percent is largely devoted to regulating when, where, and how much each protein-coding gene is expressed. Diet, stress, toxin exposure, sleep, and exercise all influence this regulatory machinery—which is the biological basis of epigenetics.

What is Epigenetics?

Epigenetics—literally "above genetics"—refers to changes in gene activity that occur without any change to the underlying DNA sequence. The most studied mechanism is DNA methylation: chemical tags that attach to DNA and switch genes on or off. These tags are not permanent; they respond dynamically to the environment. The most dramatic demonstration of epigenetics in humans is identical twins. Twins begin life with identical DNA, but by middle age, their epigenetic profiles can differ substantially—shaped by decades of different diets, stress levels, relationships, and exposures. Their genes are identical. Their gene expression is not. Epigenetic changes can also be inherited: the experiences of parents and even grandparents can leave molecular marks that influence the biology of their descendants. On the positive side, lifestyle choices—caloric moderation, regular exercise, stress management—appear to produce favorable epigenetic modifications that support longevity.

Smoking, chronic stress, and poor diet do the opposite.

How Do Genes Connect to Illness?

It is tempting to look for a single gene responsible for a disease, but most common illnesses are polygenic—the product of dozens, hundreds, or even thousands of genetic variants interacting with each other and with the environment. Schizophrenia, for instance, involves an estimated 300 or more genes, none of which is either necessary or sufficient on its own. At the other end of the spectrum, rare single-gene disorders like cystic fibrosis illustrate how precise the relationship can be: the deletion of just three DNA letters disrupts a single protein, causing it to misfold, which triggers the cascading lung and digestive damage of the disease. BRCA1 and BRCA2 sit somewhere in between: they are single genes whose mutations dramatically raise the risk of breast and ovarian cancer—but even carriers do not inevitably develop cancer. Genetic risk is probability, not fate.

Genetic Screening

Genetic screening during pregnancy focuses primarily on recessive conditions—disorders like cystic fibrosis, sickle cell disease, and Tay-Sachs disease, which only manifest when a child inherits two defective copies of the gene, one from each parent. Because both parents must be carriers, these conditions are relatively rare. Dominant genetic disorders, where a single defective copy causes disease, are generally screened for only when there is a specific family history. The most clinically important example for adults is cancer risk: anyone with a family history of cancer diagnosed at an unusually young age, or multiple relatives with the same cancer type, should consider genetic counseling and testing for high-risk genes such as BRCA1 and BRCA2. Knowing you carry a high-risk variant is not a diagnosis—it is an opportunity to monitor more aggressively and intervene earlier.

What Is CRISPR?

CRISPR-Cas9 is the most precise gene-editing tool ever developed. It functions like molecular scissors, cutting DNA at a specific location with extraordinary accuracy and enabling scientists to delete, repair, or insert genetic material. For single-gene disorders, this precision is transformative. The first CRISPR-based cure for sickle cell disease was approved in 2023, offering patients the prospect of a one-time treatment that eliminates the disease entirely. The cost—currently around $2.2 million per patient—remains a profound barrier, but the therapeutic proof of concept is now established. For complex conditions like heart disease, diabetes, and most cancers—which involve hundreds of genes interacting with environmental factors—CRISPR offers less, at least for now.

In cancer treatment, a powerful immunotherapy approach called CAR-T therapy has produced striking early results, particularly in blood cancers: a patient's own immune cells are removed, reprogrammed to recognize and attack their specific cancer, and reinfused into the bloodstream. CRISPR is now being investigated to advance CAR-T further—for example, by creating "off-the-shelf" versions that do not require harvesting the patient's own cells. The ethical frontier, however, is the modification of DNA in sperm, eggs, or early embryos, which would permanently alter every cell in all future descendants. This possibility raises profound questions about the line between treating disease and engineering human characteristics. The scientific community has broadly called for a moratorium on heritable germline editing until the safety, ethics, and governance frameworks are firmly established.

How Protein Folding Affects Health

Proteins do not work simply by existing—they must fold into precise three-dimensional shapes to perform their functions. A protein of just 100 amino acids can theoretically assume more configurations than there are atoms in the universe, yet biological proteins fold correctly in milliseconds. A landmark AI (artificial intelligence) discovery called AlphaFold, developed by Google DeepMind, has predicted the three-dimensional structures of hundreds of millions of proteins—a scientific achievement that is accelerating structural biology research and holds significant promise for drug discovery (see Chapter 20).

When proteins do not fold correctly—through mutation, environmental stress, or simple error—the results can be catastrophic. Misfolded proteins are strongly implicated in Alzheimer's disease and Parkinson's—abnormal protein aggregates are a hallmark of both conditions. In cystic fibrosis, a misfolded protein directly causes the thick mucus accumulation that damages the lungs.

Genetics, AI, and the Future of Health Care

The convergence of genomics (the entire library of genes) and artificial intelligence is opening possibilities in medicine that were unimaginable a decade ago. AI systems can now analyze a tumor's complete genetic profile and identify the specific mutations driving its growth—allowing oncologists to match patients with targeted therapies rather than generic chemotherapy. Polygenic risk scores, which aggregate the effects of hundreds of genetic variants, are increasingly being used to predict individual susceptibility to conditions like cardiovascular disease, diabetes, and Alzheimer's—enabling earlier intervention for the highest-risk individuals. AlphaFold's protein structure predictions are advancing our understanding of molecular targets—an important step toward accelerating drug discovery. The direction is clear: genetics and AI together are moving medicine from population-level treatment toward genuinely personalized care.

Conclusion

The title of this chapter is its most important message: genes are not destiny. The common diseases that shorten and diminish most lives—heart disease, stroke, diabetes, dementia, most cancers—are not determined by genetics alone. They emerge from decades of interaction between a genetic predisposition and a lived environment. That environment is largely within your control. Exercise, diet, sleep, stress management, and social connection do not merely influence your risk in some vague, general sense—they physically alter the epigenetic marks on your DNA, changing which genes are expressed and which are silenced. Meanwhile, CRISPR and AI are beginning to offer tools for the cases where genetics does play a decisive role. The future of medicine is more personal, more precise, and more hopeful than the fatalistic view of genes-as-destiny would suggest. Even from a genetic standpoint, the most powerful tool available for a longer, healthier life remains the lifestyle choices discussed throughout this book.

Chapter 9:

Lifestyle Choices Can Reduce Your Cancer Risk

CANCER IS THE DIAGNOSIS most people fear above all others. But the fear often comes packaged with a fatalistic assumption: that cancer is written in your genes, largely beyond your control, something that either happens to you or doesn't. The evidence says otherwise. Genetics accounts for only 5 to 10 percent of cancer cases. The other 90 to 95 percent arise from factors that are, to varying degrees, modifiable. Cancer death rates in the United States have fallen by roughly 30 percent since 1990—a remarkable public health achievement driven partly by better treatments, but also by the cumulative effect of lifestyle change, earlier detection, and vaccination. The World Health Organization estimates that 30 to 50 percent of all cancers could be prevented by targeting modifiable risk factors: smoking, obesity, alcohol, UV exposure, physical inactivity, and certain infections. This chapter explains what those risk factors are and what you can actually do about them.

Diet

Diet shapes cancer risk through multiple pathways: inflammation, insulin signaling, hormone levels, gut microbiome composition, and the direct effects of specific compounds on cell growth and DNA repair. A Mediterranean diet—centered on vegetables, fruits, legumes, whole grains, fatty fish, nuts, and olive oil—is associated with meaningfully lower cancer risk across multiple cancer types. Fiber is particularly well-studied: high fiber intake is consistently linked to reduced colorectal cancer risk. At the other end of the spectrum, processed and red meats are classified as carcinogens (cancer-promoting compounds) by the World Health Organization—processed meats in the highest-risk category, red meat in the category of probable carcinogen. High-sugar diets and ultra-processed foods drive chronic inflammation and insulin resistance, both of which create biological environments that favor cancer cell growth. The dietary changes most supported by evidence are the same ones that protect the heart and brain: less processed food, more plants.

Alcohol May Promote Cancer

Alcohol is a Group 1 carcinogen—the highest risk classification used by the International Agency for Research on Cancer, placing it alongside tobacco and asbestos. This is not a fringe position; it is the established scientific consensus. Alcohol increases the risk of cancers of the mouth, throat, larynx, esophagus, liver, breast, colon, and rectum. The risk is dose-dependent: it begins at low levels of consumption and rises with each additional drink. Women face significantly elevated all-cause mortality risk above about 2 drinks per day. Men's all-cause mortality risk rises meaningfully above approximately 3 to 4 drinks per day. The popular belief that moderate red wine consumption is protective for the heart—and by extension perhaps for cancer—has been substantially revised by more recent research that accounted for confounding factors—for example, people who drink wine daily tend to have better healthcare access and less stressful jobs. For cancer prevention specifically, there is no established safe level of alcohol.

Quit Smoking to Prevent Cancers

Smoking is the single most powerful preventable cause of cancer in the world. It is responsible for approximately 90 percent of all lung cancers—still the leading cancer killer in the United States—but its damage extends far beyond the lungs. Smoking increases risk for cancers of the larynx, esophagus, bladder, pancreas, cervix, kidney, stomach, liver, colon, and blood (acute myeloid leukemia). Secondhand smoke is not a minor concern: it raises lung cancer risk in non-smokers by 20 to 30 percent, has been linked to elevated breast cancer risk in premenopausal women, and affects children's cancer risk as well. The biology of recovery after quitting is genuinely encouraging: within ten years of stopping, a former smoker's lung cancer risk falls to roughly half that of a current smoker; within 15 to 20 years, it approaches the risk of someone who never smoked. Quitting at any age reduces risk. The earlier, the better.

Body Weight and Cancer

The cancer risk from excess body weight is substantially underappreciated—by patients and, often, by physicians. Adipose (fat) tissue is not merely a passive energy store; it is metabolically active, producing hormones (particularly estrogen and insulin) and chronic inflammatory signals that promote cell proliferation and tumor growth. A landmark UK study of 1.2 million women found striking associations between higher body weight and multiple cancer types. Across large U.S. and international studies, obesity accounts for approximately 11 percent of cancers in women and 5 percent in men. The evidence for intervention is also encouraging: bariatric surgery reduces overall cancer incidence in severely obese patients, and women who intentionally lose at least 10 percent of their body weight show a measurably lower risk of breast cancer.

Physical Activity

Regular physical activity is one of the most robustly documented cancer-protective behaviors. Large-scale studies consistently find that more active individuals have lower rates of colon, breast, and endometrial cancer—three of the most common cancer types—with risk reductions in the range of 20 to 40 percent compared to the most sedentary individuals. The mechanisms are multiple: exercise reduces circulating estrogen and insulin, both of which fuel hormone-sensitive cancers; it lowers chronic inflammation, which drives DNA damage and tumor-promoting signaling; and it directly helps maintain a healthy body weight. For people already diagnosed with cancer, exercise is no longer a passive recommendation—it is now endorsed by major oncology organizations as part of treatment, improving response rates, reducing treatment-related side effects, and improving survival in some cancer types. Both aerobic activity and resistance training contribute, and the benefits appear to begin at modest activity levels, increasing with greater intensity and duration.

Sun Exposure

Skin cancer is the most commonly diagnosed cancer in the United States, and ultraviolet radiation—from sun exposure and tanning beds—is its primary cause. UV radiation damages DNA in skin cells, and the risk accumulates with every unprotected exposure over a lifetime. Melanoma, the deadliest form, is strongly associated with intense, intermittent sun exposure and blistering sunburns, particularly in childhood. Squamous and basal cell carcinomas are driven more by cumulative lifetime exposure. Protection is straightforward and effective: use a broad-spectrum sunscreen with SPF 30 or higher, apply it generously and reapply every two hours when outdoors, wear protective clothing including hats and UV-blocking fabrics, seek shade during peak UV hours (10 a.m. to 4 p.m.), and avoid UV tanning devices entirely—indoor tanning increases melanoma risk by 75 percent when first used before age 35. The cosmetic benefits of sun protection—reduced wrinkles, sunspots, and skin aging—are a bonus.

Infections and Cancer

Approximately 13 percent of all cancers worldwide are caused by infectious agents—a proportion that is almost entirely preventable. Human papillomavirus (HPV) is the most consequential: it causes virtually all cervical cancers, as well as a growing proportion of throat, anal, vaginal, vulvar, and penile cancers. The HPV vaccine, when administered before a person becomes sexually active, is nearly 100 percent effective at preventing the HPV strains responsible for most cervical cancers. Current guidelines recommend vaccination for all adolescents, and it is now approved through age 45 for those not previously vaccinated. Regular Pap smears and HPV testing remain essential for sexually active women, detecting precancerous changes years before they become invasive cancer. Hepatitis B vaccination substantially reduces the risk of hepatocellular (liver) cancer, one of the deadliest and fastest-growing cancers globally. Screening for and eradicating Helicobacter pylori—a bacterial infection of the stomach lining—can prevent the majority of stomach cancers attributable to this pathogen. This test and treatment should be considered if you or family members have a history of stomach cancer or ulcers and if you have persistent indigestion. There are some racial groups that have a higher risk (i.e., from Eastern Europe and East Asia), and this should be discussed with your medical provider.

Cancer Screening

Early detection saves lives, and the appropriate screening strategy depends on your individual risk profile. For breast cancer, mammography screening guidelines have recently been updated, with screening recommended starting at age 40 for average-risk women. The American Cancer Society formally recommends annual screening from age 45 (with the option to start at 40–44), transitioning to every two years after 55, continuing as long as overall health is good and life expectancy exceeds ten years. Given the increasing rate of breast cancer in women in their 40s—and the particularly high mortality burden in Black women, who have a 40 percent higher death rate from breast cancer than white women—discuss the right starting age with your physician rather than waiting for guidelines to fully settle. Women with BRCA1 or BRCA2 mutations should begin screening earlier, typically with annual MRI in addition to mammography. For women with dense breast tissue, 3D mammography improves detection. Family history of cancer diagnosed at a young age, or multiple relatives with the same cancer, is an indication for genetic counseling and possible BRCA or Lynch syndrome (an inherited genetic condition that increases cancer risk) testing. Annual low-dose CT scan is recommended for adults aged 50 to 80 with a 20 pack year smoking history who currently smoke or have quit within the last 15 years.

Pollution and Workplace Carcinogens

Environmental carcinogens—both outdoor and occupational—account for a meaningful proportion of cancer burden, particularly for people who live near industrial sites or work in high-exposure settings. Outdoor air pollution, including vehicle exhaust, industrial emissions, and wildfire smoke, has been classified as a Group 1 carcinogen and is linked to lung cancer even in non-smokers. In heavily polluted areas or during wildfire events, N95 masks provide meaningful protection. Occupational exposures to asbestos, benzene, formaldehyde, arsenic, cadmium, chromium, and vinyl chloride are associated with cancers of the lung, bladder, blood, and skin. Workers in high-exposure industries—construction, mining, chemical manufacturing, painting—should use appropriate respirators and protective clothing, and should be aware of their right to exposure information under workplace safety regulations. Indoor radon—a naturally occurring radioactive gas that seeps from soil into homes—is the second leading cause of lung cancer in the United States after smoking; homes in high-risk areas should be tested; if levels are elevated, consult with experts to remove the source.

Conclusion

Cancer is not, for most people, a matter of genetic fate. The choices described in this chapter—not smoking, limiting alcohol, maintaining a healthy weight, exercising regularly, protecting skin from UV, vaccinating against HPV and hepatitis B, screening appropriately, and minimizing exposure to known carcinogens—collectively address the vast majority of modifiable cancer risk. None of these interventions is exotic or expensive. Most are the same lifestyle changes that protect the heart, brain, and metabolic health described in earlier chapters. Preventing cancer is not a separate project from maximizing your health span and lifespan—it is part of the same project.

SECTION TWO

A System-by-System tour of the aging body

THE NINE CHAPTERS YOU have just read make the case that most of leading causes of premature death, what shortens life is preventable. Those chapters were, by design, organized around what you can do. Section Two shifts the lens: rather than asking what interventions produce the greatest impact on lifespan, it asks what actually happens to each organ system as we age, which of those changes are inevitable, which are preventable, and what the evidence says about managing each one. The division is not absolute — blood pressure matters to your kidneys as much as to your heart, and the Mediterranean diet protects your gut as surely as your arteries. But the system-by-system tour that follows is designed to give you a practical map of your aging body: what to watch for, when to act, and what your options are.

Chapter 10:

Your Muscles, Bones, and Joints

FEW ASPECTS OF AGING are more universally felt than what happens to the musculoskeletal system. Joints stiffen, muscles shrink, bones quietly hollow out. Most people assume these changes are simply the price of getting older—inevitable, unmanageable, best endured. The science tells a more useful story. While some musculoskeletal change is unavoidable, its pace and severity are heavily influenced by choices you make every day. The decisions described in this chapter—about exercise, diet, fall prevention, and when to pursue treatment—can preserve your strength, protect your independence, and keep you moving decades longer than inactivity would allow.

Avoid Injuries — Crucial for Health Span and Lifespan

As bones and joints age, injury risk rises sharply. Each year, one in four older adults will experience a fall, and by age 85, nearly half will fall at least once per year. Falls account for 95 percent of hip fractures—injuries that frequently lead to prolonged hospitalization, lasting loss of independence, and a cascade of physical decline. Preventing falls begins at home. Install grab bars in bathrooms, use handrails on staircases, and keep all walkways well-lit. Remove trip hazards from floors, wear supportive shoes rather than socks on smooth surfaces, rearrange furniture to open clear paths, and keep frequently used items within easy reach. On wet or icy surfaces, slow down and pay attention. If a cane or walking aid makes you steadier, use it without hesitation—it is a tool, not a concession. Review your medications with your physician: many drugs affect balance, including sedatives, blood pressure medications, and antihistamines. When rising from a seated or lying position, move slowly—orthostatic hypotension (a sudden drop in blood pressure when standing) is a common and underappreciated cause of falls, especially in older adults on blood pressure medications.

Exercises to Decrease Fall Risk and Keep Bones and Joints Healthy

Regular exercise—particularly strength training and balance work, described in detail in Chapter 1—is the single most effective intervention for reducing fall risk. Stronger muscles stabilize joints and absorb impact. Better balance prevents the stumbles that become falls. Walking, stretching, yoga, and tai chi all contribute. When starting a new exercise program, increase intensity and duration gradually; abrupt jumps in load are how injuries happen. Maintaining a healthy weight matters here too: every pound of excess body weight adds roughly four pounds of force to the knee joint with each step. The joint that seemed manageable at one weight can become a daily source of pain at another.

Osteoarthritis (OA)

Osteoarthritis (OA) is the most common form of arthritis and the most prevalent joint disease worldwide. As we age, the cartilage that cushions our joints gradually thins and breaks down. Less cartilage and less joint fluid means stiffer, less flexible joints—particularly in the knees, hips, and spine. Eventually, bone surfaces begin to contact each other, generating the characteristic pain and grinding sensation of advanced OA. Other symptoms include morning stiffness that eases with movement, reduced range of motion, and the development of bony spurs around affected joints that can feel like hard lumps under the skin. OA does not have to be a sentence of progressive pain. The choices that follow make a real difference.

Risk Factors for OA

Excess body weight is the most modifiable major risk factor for OA. The mechanical load it places on weight-bearing joints accelerates cartilage breakdown over years and decades. Family history increases susceptibility, and women develop OA more frequently than men—particularly after menopause, when declining estrogen levels may reduce cartilage protection. Previous joint injuries, even ones that healed well, leave joints more vulnerable to OA later in life. Using proper form during physical activity, wearing supportive footwear, and staying active all meaningfully reduce OA risk. Low-impact exercise—swimming, cycling, walking—is particularly valuable because it strengthens surrounding muscles and nourishes cartilage through joint fluid circulation without the repetitive impact that wears it down.

Tendons and Ligaments

Tendons connect muscles to bones; ligaments connect bones to each other at joints. Both are fibrous connective tissues that degrade gradually with age. Tendons become stiffer and less elastic; ligaments lose elastin content, reducing flexibility and joint stability. This degeneration can accelerate cartilage wear and contribute to OA. The range of motion available at the spine, hips, and ankles tends to decline as tendons and ligaments stiffen, raising the risk of strains and tears. Healing slows significantly with age, so injuries that would have resolved in weeks at age 30 may take months at age 65. The practical implication: it becomes increasingly important with age to warm up before activity, build intensity gradually, and take soft tissue pain seriously early rather than pushing through it.

Tendinopathy

Tendon pain—tendinopathy—becomes more common with each decade, and affects roughly one in four adults at any given time. The most frequently affected areas are the rotator cuff in the shoulder, the Achilles tendon at the heel, and the lateral elbow, (commonly called tennis elbow, though most sufferers have never played tennis). Tendinopathy develops when tendons are subjected to loads that exceed their capacity to recover—either from sudden increases in activity, repetitive overuse, or age-related tissue changes. To prevent it, avoid sharp increases in the weight you lift or the intensity of your training. If you develop tendon pain that is sharp, is accompanied by swelling, or wakes you at night, see a physical therapist rather than trying to train through it. Most tendinopathy responds well to a structured rehabilitation program; ignored, it can progress to partial or complete tears that require months of recovery.

Your Muscles as You Age

Muscle is not merely cosmetic—it is the primary protector of your joints, the engine of your balance, and a major determinant of whether you remain physically independent as you age. Beginning around age 30, we lose approximately 3 to 8 percent of muscle mass per decade, with the rate of loss accelerating significantly after age 60. This condition is called sarcopenia, and it is far more consequential than its quiet progression suggests. Sarcopenic adults fall more often, recover from illness more slowly, and lose independence earlier than those who maintain muscle mass. The underlying biology involves declining levels of testosterone and growth hormone, reduced protein synthesis efficiency, and increasing inflammatory signaling. All of these age-related changes can be countered by regular exercise. Weakness in the quadriceps (the large muscles at the front of the thigh) is one of the strongest predictors of knee pain and progression of knee OA, because strong quads offload the joint. Preserving them is both a strategy for mobility and a strategy for pain management.

How to Decrease / Prevent Muscle Loss

The most effective intervention for sarcopenia is resistance training—and it works at virtually any age. Studies in adults in their 80s and 90s have demonstrated meaningful gains in muscle mass and strength from structured programs, with corresponding improvements in balance and function. Aim for strength training two to three times per week, progressively increasing resistance as you get stronger. Free weights, machines, resistance bands, and bodyweight exercises (push-ups, lunges, squats, pull-ups) all work. Diet matters alongside exercise: adequate protein intake is essential for muscle protein synthesis. Include lean meats, fish, eggs, legumes, and dairy regularly, and consider distributing protein intake across meals rather than concentrating it in one sitting. One important caution: GLP-1 receptor agonists (such as semaglutide and tirzepatide), increasingly used for weight loss, can cause significant muscle loss alongside fat loss—particularly without accompanying resistance training (see chapter 2). Older adults taking these medications should prioritize protein intake and strength training to preserve the muscle mass they cannot afford to lose.

Bone Health / Osteoporosis

Bone density peaks in the late twenties to early thirties, then begins a slow decline. After age 35, bone breakdown begins to outpace bone formation. In many people, this progression reaches the threshold of osteoporosis—bones so porous that ordinary activities like coughing, bending, or stepping off a curb can cause fractures. Many individuals lose up to a third of their peak bone density by age 70. Osteoporosis earns its description as a silent disease: it produces no symptoms until a fracture occurs. Women face accelerated bone loss after menopause as estrogen levels fall, but men are by no means immune—approximately one in four men over 50 will have an osteoporosis-related fracture in their lifetime. The most consequential fracture sites are the wrist, hip, and spine. A hip fracture triggers a chain of consequences—surgery, immobility, deconditioning, loss of independence—that many older adults never fully recover from. Spinal compression fractures cause progressive height loss and the forward-stooping posture known as kyphosis.

Preventing / Treating Osteoporosis

Exercise remains the cornerstone of osteoporosis prevention. Weight-bearing and resistance exercise—walking, stair climbing, strength training—apply mechanical stress to bone that stimulates new bone formation. Avoid smoking, which directly accelerates bone loss, and limit alcohol consumption for the same reason. Adequate calcium and vitamin D intake is essential: older adults generally need around 1,000 to 1,200 mg of calcium daily through diet and supplementation, and 800 to 1,000 IU of vitamin D3 to ensure absorption. Adequate protein intake supports bone matrix as well as muscle. Bone density scanning (DEXA) is recommended for all women at age 65, earlier for those with risk factors such as low body weight, long-term steroid use, smoking, or excessive alcohol use. Men should be screened at age 70, or earlier with risk factors. When bone density is significantly low, effective medications are available. A weekly oral bisphosphonate (alendronate, brand name Fosamax) or a once-yearly intravenous infusion (zoledronic acid, brand name Reclast) can meaningfully reduce fracture risk by slowing bone breakdown. Hormone replacement therapy may also reduce bone loss in postmenopausal women—discussed further in Chapter 12.

Non-Surgical Management of Joint Pain

For older adults with mild to moderate joint pain, conservative treatment is always the appropriate first approach. Physical therapy to strengthen the muscles surrounding a painful joint is among the most effective interventions available—and among the most underused. Over-the-counter options include NSAIDs such as ibuprofen (Advil, Motrin) or naproxen (Aleve, Naprosyn), and acetaminophen (Tylenol). NSAIDs are more effective anti-inflammatory agents but carry risks with prolonged use, particularly for the stomach, kidneys, and cardiovascular system; use the lowest effective dose for the shortest necessary period. When these approaches fall short, corticosteroid injections directly into the joint can provide meaningful short-term relief, particularly for knee OA. Hyaluronic acid (HA) injections are another option—generally safer for repeated use than steroids, and capable of providing modest pain relief and improved function, though their effect compared to placebo is not dramatic. Platelet-rich plasma (PRP) injections—prepared from your own blood and injected into the joint to promote healing—may provide longer-lasting relief than either HA or steroid injections for knee arthritis in some patients, though cost is high and insurance coverage is inconsistent.

Exercise as a Treatment for Osteoarthritis

For many years, patients with severe OA were advised to rest and avoid activity that might "wear out" the joint further. Current evidence has reversed that thinking entirely. Exercise is now recognized as one of the most effective non-surgical treatments for OA, even in severe cases where x-rays show bone-on-bone contact. A structured exercise program developed with a physical therapist reduces pain, maintains joint fluid circulation (which nourishes cartilage and prevents the joint capsule from stiffening), and—critically—strengthens the quadriceps and surrounding muscles, which take mechanical load off the damaged joint surface. Weak quadriceps are one of the most consistent predictors of knee pain progression; strengthening them is a direct therapeutic intervention. High-impact activities can worsen OA and should be avoided, but the answer is not to stop moving—it is to choose the right kind of movement. Work with a physical therapist to design a program appropriate for your specific joint and degree of involvement.

Surgical Orthopedic Options

Before agreeing to any elective orthopedic surgery, I strongly recommend getting a second opinion from an independent orthopedic surgeon—not a partner or associate of the first—to confirm that surgery is genuinely the best option and that non-surgical alternatives have been adequately explored. Physical therapy, medications, injections, and lifestyle modification can eliminate or substantially reduce symptoms in many patients who are initially told surgery is their only path forward. When surgery is being considered, understand the specific risks: infection, blood clots, nerve injury, implant failure, and the possibility of incomplete pain relief. Discuss realistic outcomes with your surgeon before consenting, not after.

Low Back Pain

Back pain is one of the most economically and personally costly health conditions in the world. In the United States, Americans spend more treating chronic pain than treating diabetes and cancer combined. Low back pain is now the single leading cause of years lived with disability globally—surpassing all other conditions—and is one of the most common reasons for opioid prescriptions in the U.S., contributing significantly to the ongoing opioid crisis. A combination of physical therapy, targeted spinal injections, and non-opioid pain medications can successfully manage most cases without surgery. For mild to moderate pain, physical therapy is the appropriate first treatment. Epidural (lower back, along spine) corticosteroid injections can provide meaningful short-term relief when physical therapy alone is insufficient. Non-opioid medications including NSAIDs (ibuprofen, naproxen), and muscle relaxants such as cyclobenzaprine (Flexeril) can help manage acute flare-ups. Surgery is reserved for severe cases where conservative treatment has genuinely failed, but it does not guarantee full pain relief or return to normal function. In fact, for lumbar disc herniation specifically, multiple clinical trials—including the landmark SPORT trial—have found no significant difference in outcomes at one to two years between patients who had surgery and those who received aggressive conservative care. This is not a reason to avoid surgery when it is truly indicated; it is a reason to exhaust non-surgical options first.

My own encounter with this is worth sharing. More than twenty years ago, a lumbar disc herniation kept me out of work for nearly a month with severe sciatica. I was aware of the research showing no significant long-term advantage for surgery over conservative care—the same evidence the SPORT trial would later confirm—and I chose to wait, managing with physical therapy, spinal injections, and medication. What I did not fully appreciate at the time was how much my pain was being amplified by something beyond the disc itself. I was in the middle of a deeply stressful personal situation, and I believe that sustained emotional conflict kept my nervous system in a state of heightened threat response—which, as the section below describes, directly lowers the threshold at which the brain generates pain signals. The disc was real. The injury was real. But the intensity and duration of my pain were shaped by more than anatomy. I have been essentially free of sciatica since, and I attribute that not to the treatments I received during that episode but to what came after: better sleep, lower chronic stress, and a daily commitment to exercise and stretching.

The Psychology and Neuroscience of Chronic Pain

One of the most important—and most underused—tools for managing chronic pain requires no prescription, no procedure, and no referral to a surgeon. It requires understanding what chronic pain actually is. For decades, pain was understood as a simple signal: tissue is damaged, nerves fire, the brain receives a warning. This model works reasonably well for acute pain. It fails for chronic pain. When pain persists for months or years—

especially after the original injury has healed or in the absence of any identifiable structural cause—something fundamentally different is happening. The nervous system itself has changed. In a process called central sensitization, the brain and spinal cord become hyperexcitable: pain pathways that were activated repeatedly begin firing more easily, at lower thresholds, and in response to stimuli that would not normally be painful. The alarm system has been turned up. This is not imagined pain—the neurological changes are real and measurable—but the driver of the pain is now in the nervous system's processing, not in the tissue itself. This distinction matters enormously, because it means that interventions aimed only at the tissue—another injection, another surgery, another round of opioids—are addressing the wrong target. What changes the nervous system is different from what changes a disc or a joint.

Several non-pharmacological approaches have meaningful evidence for reducing chronic pain. Structured programs teach patients what central sensitization is, why pain is not always a reliable signal of tissue damage, and how the nervous system's threat perception drives pain intensity. This approach, particularly when combined with exercise and physical therapy, consistently reduces both pain and pain-related disability. The mechanism is cognitive: patients who understand that movement is not inherently dangerous become less fearful of it, engage more fully in physical therapy, and break the cycle of avoidance that deepens deconditioning and worsens pain over time. Cognitive behavioral therapy (CBT) for chronic pain targets the thinking patterns—catastrophizing, hypervigilance, helplessness—that amplify pain signals and impair function. CBT does not eliminate pain, but it meaningfully reduces pain interference with daily life and improves physical functioning and mood. Mindfulness-based stress reduction, non-judgmental awareness of physical sensation, produces comparable outcomes to CBT for chronic low back pain. Sleep has a bidirectional relationship with chronic pain that is frequently overlooked: inadequate sleep lowers pain thresholds, and chronic pain disrupts sleep, creating a reinforcing cycle. Addressing sleep through behavioral interventions often reduces pain independent of other treatment. Social connection and meaningful activity matter too: isolation and loss of purpose, both common in older adults with chronic pain, independently amplify pain perception. None of these approaches replaces physical therapy, appropriate medication, or well-indicated procedures.

Orthopedic Procedures of Questionable Value

Not all orthopedic procedures deliver the outcomes patients expect. Several widely performed surgeries have been shown in rigorous trials to be no more effective than conservative management—and in some cases less effective. Arthroscopic debridement for knee osteoarthritis, which involves cleaning the joint and removing loose tissue, has not demonstrated meaningful benefit over physical therapy and strengthening exercises in patients with degenerative OA. Surgical repair of small or partial rotator cuff tears often produces outcomes no better than physical therapy and activity modification, which should be exhausted before surgical repair is pursued. For mild to moderate carpal tunnel syndrome—which causes tingling, numbness, and the sensation of a 'hand falling asleep' in the thumb, index, middle, and part of the ring finger—splinting, steroid injections, and targeted therapy are frequently effective and should precede surgical release. Surgical treatment of lateral epicondylitis (tennis elbow) and shoulder tendinosis has not shown significantly better outcomes than non-surgical treatment in mild to moderate cases. Spinal fusion for chronic degenerative disc disease, in many cases, produces outcomes comparable to—or no better than—physical therapy, exercise, and pain management. This is not to say surgery is never appropriate, but the decision should be made with a clear-eyed understanding of what the evidence shows.

When Surgery Makes Sense

Surgery becomes the right choice when joint pain is severe enough to substantially impair daily life and has not responded to a genuine, sustained trial of conservative treatment. Joint replacement—most commonly of the hip, knee, or shoulder—can be transformative for patients with end-stage arthritis. Modern prostheses typically last 15 to 20 years, providing dramatic pain relief and restoration of function for the right candidates. Recovery requires patience: return to full activity generally takes three to six months, and the rehabilitation process demands real effort. The risks—infection, blood clot, implant failure, nerve injury—are real and should be discussed candidly. For appropriately selected patients who have done the work of conservative management first, joint replacement is among the most reliably successful procedures in medicine.

Conclusion

The musculoskeletal changes of aging—cartilage thinning, bone loss, muscle wasting, tendon stiffening—are real, but they are not fixed in their trajectory. The patients I have watched age most successfully share a common profile: they kept moving, they kept lifting, they ate enough protein, they protected their joints from unnecessary injury. When pain does arise, the evidence consistently favors conservative management over early surgery, and an understanding of the science of chronic pain. The conditions described in this chapter—osteoarthritis, sarcopenia, osteoporosis, tendinopathy—respond to lifestyle choices more than almost any other organ system in the body. Exercise — specifically resistance training combined with balance and aerobic work — is the single most powerful intervention available for every condition covered in this chapter.

Chapter 11:

Understanding Skin Care and Hair Health as We Age

THE ANTI-AGING SKINCARE INDUSTRY is one of the largest and fastest-growing consumer markets in the world, currently valued in the tens of billions of dollars and expanding every year. This scale reflects a genuine human concern—the visible changes aging brings to skin and hair are among the first signs of getting older, and they are hard to ignore. But the size of an industry is not evidence of its effectiveness. In this chapter, I will distinguish the small number of topical interventions supported by real evidence from the far larger category of products sold on hope, marketing, and the placebo effect. A focused, evidence-based approach to skin and hair care is not only more effective than indiscriminate product use—it is also considerably cheaper.

Skin and Hair Changes With Age

As we age, the skin undergoes predictable structural changes. Collagen production declines—beginning as early as the mid-twenties and accelerating with age—causing the dermis (the true skin containing the live components, as opposed to the epidermis, the top layer made up mostly of dead protective cells) to thin and lose structural support. Elastin fibers degrade, reducing the skin's ability to spring back, leading to sagging and deeper wrinkles. Sebaceous glands become less active, reducing natural oil production and contributing to the dry, sometimes itchy skin that many older adults notice. Sun exposure accelerates all of these changes by generating oxidative damage that degrades collagen and stimulates melanin irregularities (age spots). In hair follicles, depletion of melanin leads to gray hair. Understanding these mechanisms helps explain why certain ingredients—retinoids, antioxidants, and sunscreen—are worth using, and why so many others are not.

Effective Skin Care Products

Many over-the-counter skincare products claim anti-aging effects, but the evidence supporting most of them is limited. The FDA regulates cosmetics differently from drugs: a cosmetic product does not need to demonstrate efficacy before reaching the market. The clinical studies that do exist for OTC products are frequently industry-funded, short-term, conducted in small samples, and not independently replicated. The placebo effect is also meaningful in skincare—when people expect a cream to work and pay a premium for it, they perceive improvement that may not correspond to measurable change. Among the most common and most misleading ingredients in premium anti-aging products are topical collagen and elastin. Both molecules are far too large to penetrate the skin's outer layer; they may temporarily improve texture through surface hydration, but they cannot rebuild the collagen or elastin network beneath the skin. Peptides have a more plausible mechanism but limited evidence of meaningful clinical effect at OTC concentrations. The ingredients that do have solid evidence—retinoids, sunscreen, hyaluronic acid, niacinamide, and vitamin C—are discussed below.

Sunscreen

Sunscreen is not merely a cancer-prevention product—it is the single most evidence-based anti-photoaging topical intervention available without a prescription. (Photoaging refers to skin damage caused by sun exposure, as distinct from the natural aging process.) Decades of UV sun exposure is the leading cause of wrinkles, sunspots, loss of elasticity, and uneven skin tone rather than the natural aging process alone. Daily sunscreen use has been shown in randomized controlled trials to reduce photoaging and new sunspots compared to unprotected skin. Use a broad-spectrum SPF 30 or higher daily—'broad spectrum' is essential because SPF values measure only UVB protection, while UVA rays penetrate more deeply and cause destructive changes in the dermis. Apply it as the final step in your morning routine, after other active ingredients. Protective clothing, hats with wide brims, and avoiding peak sun hours (10 a.m. to 2 p.m.) compound the benefit. If you use nothing else from this chapter, use sunscreen daily.

Retinoids

Retinoids—derivatives of vitamin A—are the most rigorously studied topical ingredients for aging skin and among the very few with robust evidence of genuine benefit. The active form, retinoic acid, works by activating genes that stimulate collagen and elastin synthesis in the dermis. Retinoids also accelerate cell turnover in the epidermis, which thickens the skin, reduces fine lines, and fades sun damage over time. There is a potency hierarchy worth understanding: retinol (the most common OTC form) must be converted to retinoic acid by skin enzymes, making it less potent but better tolerated; retinaldehyde is a more direct precursor and somewhat stronger; tretinoin (prescription only) is the direct active form—the most potent and most extensively studied. Prescription tretinoin produces the most reliable results but requires medical oversight. OTC retinoids are genuinely effective, though they work more slowly. Because retinoids cause sun sensitivity and can cause significant irritation when first introduced, start with a low concentration two to three nights per week and increase frequency gradually as tolerance builds. Pairing with a hydrating product like hyaluronic acid reduces irritation. Retinoids are contraindicated during pregnancy and should be stopped when trying to conceive.

Hyaluronic Acid

Hyaluronic acid (HA) is a glycosaminoglycan—a naturally occurring molecule in the skin's connective tissue—that can hold up to 1,000 times its weight in water. When applied topically, it draws moisture to the skin's surface, temporarily reducing the appearance of fine lines and restoring a plumper, more hydrated look. Because HA molecules are often too large to penetrate deeply into the skin, products formulated with multiple molecular weights (both high and low) provide more complete surface and sub-surface hydration than single-weight products. One practical consideration: in very low-humidity environments, high-molecular-weight HA may draw moisture from deeper skin layers rather than from the air, potentially increasing dryness. Applying HA to slightly damp skin and following with a moisturizer or occlusive layer helps seal in hydration. HA is well-tolerated by virtually all skin types, making it one of the easiest active ingredients to incorporate into a routine.

Niacinamide (Vitamin B3)

Niacinamide (vitamin B3) is one of the most broadly useful and best-tolerated active ingredients in skincare. It strengthens the skin barrier by stimulating the synthesis of lipid molecules that hold skin cells together and prevent water loss. It reduces skin darkening and helps even skin tone without the irritation associated with other agents. Its anti-inflammatory action calms redness and helps manage the inflammation underlying conditions like rosacea and acne. It also regulates skin oil production, making it valuable for oily or acne-prone skin. Niacinamide is compatible with essentially all other skincare products and offers meaningful benefit with little risk.

Vitamin C (L-Ascorbic Acid)

Vitamin C (L-ascorbic acid) is one of the best-studied antioxidants in skincare. Antioxidants interrupt the chemical reactions that damage cellular structures and proteins, which in the skin translates to protection against the oxidative damage caused by UV radiation and environmental pollutants. Vitamin C also plays a direct role in collagen synthesis and inhibits melanin production, helping to fade existing dark spots and prevent new ones. L-ascorbic acid is the most bioactive and most studied form, but it has a significant practical limitation: it oxidizes rapidly on exposure to air, light, and heat, turning yellow or orange and losing efficacy. A product that has changed color has likely lost most of its potency. For stability, L-ascorbic acid requires packaging that minimizes air exposure—pumps or tubes rather than open jars. Apply in the morning before sunscreen for added UV protection.

Combining Skincare Ingredients

Layering skincare ingredients in the right order improves both efficacy and tolerability. In the morning, apply a cleanser, then hyaluronic acid (while skin is slightly damp), then your vitamin C , and finish with broad-spectrum SPF 30+ sunscreen (which can also serve as moisturizer). In the evening, cleanse, apply hyaluronic acid, then niacinamide, then your retinoid, and finish with a moisturizer to buffer any retinoid irritation. Retinoids are best used at night: UV exposure degrades retinoic acid on contact, and cell turnover peaks during sleep, making evening application more effective. A common myth worth dispelling: vitamin C and niacinamide are frequently said to be incompatible, but this concern is based on outdated chemistry and is not supported by current evidence. At the concentrations used in most skincare products, they can be used together without issue. When starting a retinoid, use it only two to three nights per week initially and increase frequency as your skin adapts.

Hair Loss

Male and female pattern baldness each have two treatments with robust evidence. Topical minoxidil (available OTC as Rogaine) works in both men and women. Results are modest, variable, and dependent on continued use: stopping treatment typically results in loss of any gained hair within several months. Finasteride (Propecia) blocks production of the hormone responsible for male pattern hair loss. At one year, 48 percent of men showed improvement by photographic assessment; this rose to 66 percent at two years. However, finasteride showed no significant benefit in postmenopausal women in a placebo-controlled trial. For men, finasteride requires two important caveats: it reduces PSA levels by approximately 50 percent, which can mask early prostate cancer. In 2011, the FDA added a warning about depression to finasteride's label after reports of persistent sexual and psychological side effects (known as post-finasteride syndrome) in some users following discontinuation. A dermatologist can help determine whether treatment is appropriate and which option suits your pattern of hair loss.

Conclusion

What the evidence in this chapter shows is how disproportionate the returns are from a very short list of ingredients. Sunscreen is doing more work than everything else combined—

preventing the UV damage, the dominant driver of visible aging, reducing skin cancer risk, and protecting whatever else you apply underneath it. A retinoid, used consistently, is the only topical ingredient with strong evidence that it slows the impact of aging on your skin. Vitamin C, hyaluronic acid, and niacinamide each fill specific gaps—antioxidant protection, hydration, and barrier support—at low cost and low risk. If hair loss is a significant concern, a dermatologist is the right starting point—not the supplement aisle. And for anyone with rosacea, significant acne, pronounced photoaging, or suspicious lesions—a dermatologist can offer prescription-strength tretinoin and a biopsy of potential cancerous skin lesions.

Chapter 12:

Hormone Therapy and Aging

HORMONES ARE THE BODY'S long-range chemical messengers—secreted by glands, carried through the bloodstream, and capable of influencing virtually every tissue and organ. As we age, the production of several key hormones declines in predictable ways, and the symptoms that follow are among the most discussed—and most frequently mismanaged—aspects of aging medicine. This chapter covers three areas where the evidence is frequently misread in both directions: thyroid hormone, where the impulse to treat subclinical findings often outpaces the evidence; female sex hormones, where a flawed 2002 study caused decades of unnecessary suffering by discouraging appropriate hormone therapy; and testosterone, where both overtreatment and undertreatment are common. Sexual health and STI risk in older adults are also addressed.

Thyroid Hormones

As people age, thyroid function can decline. The most common age-related finding is subclinical hypothyroidism—defined as an elevated TSH (thyroid-stimulating hormone) with a normal free T4. Many patients and some clinicians assume this warrants treatment, but the evidence says otherwise. The TRUST trial—a randomized, placebo-controlled trial found that thyroid hormone treatment produced no improvement in symptoms, quality of life, or cognitive function compared to placebo. For most older adults with subclinical hypothyroidism, watchful waiting with periodic monitoring is the appropriate approach. Treatment carries risks including atrial fibrillation (see Chapter 4) and accelerated bone loss. True hypothyroidism (elevated TSH with low T4) is a different matter and generally warrants treatment.

Menopause

Menopause—the permanent cessation of menstrual periods—occurs at a median age of 51 in the United States. The years leading up to menopause (perimenopause) can begin a decade earlier, as estrogen and progesterone levels fluctuate and decline, producing a wide range of effects including hot flashes, night sweats, disrupted sleep, mood instability, cognitive fog, vaginal dryness, urinary urgency, and discomfort during sex that results from estrogen-dependent tissue atrophy. Hot flashes typically last four to seven years but persist beyond ten years in many women. Black and Hispanic women experience symptoms earlier, more severely, and for longer than white women on average. The decline in estrogen also accelerates bone loss (see Chapter 10) and women's cardiovascular risk rises sharply after menopause approaching that of men within a decade. Topical estrogen (cream, ring, or suppository) is the most effective treatment for the genitourinary syndrome of menopause (GSM), which includes urinary symptoms such as urgency, frequency, and burning on urination, as well as irritation and itching of the vulva, vaginal dryness, and painful intercourse.

Hormone Replacement Therapy (HRT) for Women

HRT effectively reduces hot flashes, night sweats, sleep disruption, and GSM symptoms, and meaningfully lowers the risk of bone fractures and urinary tract infections. The evidence on cardiovascular benefit is also favorable when HRT is started within ten years of menopause or before age 60 (the "timing hypothesis"): estrogen improves the lipid profile, reduces arterial inflammation, and appears to slow the progression of atherosclerosis during the window when vessels are still relatively healthy.

The breast cancer issue is a bit complicated. The 2002 Women's Health Initiative (WHI) trial alarmed clinicians and patients by reporting increased breast cancer risk with HRT. The WHI studied combined estrogen-progestogen therapy in women who were, on average, 63 years old and a decade past menopause. Critics correctly identified that this was the wrong population to draw conclusions about women initiating HRT in their early 50s. However, the breast cancer risk for combined estrogen-progestogen HRT is real. A study involving 100,000 women found a meaningful increase in risk with combined estrogen-progesterone therapy. For most women this represents a small increased risk that must be weighed individually against the substantial benefits, and that risk varies by HRT type, duration of use, and timing of initiation. The recommendation is to start HRT within ten years of menopause onset or before age

60, use the lowest effective dose, reassess the need periodically, and undergo regular mammography. For women who cannot or prefer not to use hormone therapy, non-hormonal prescription options now exist for symptoms like hot flashes and night sweats: fezolinetant (Veozah, FDA-approved 2023). This is a complex issue that you must address with your health care provider.

Andropause and Testosterone Replacement Therapy (TRT)

Men experience a gradual age-related decline in testosterone—often called andropause, though this term is less precise than "female menopause," since the decline is slow and continuous rather than abrupt. Testosterone peaks in the late teens and early twenties, then falls by roughly 1 to 2 percent of total testosterone per year after age 30 to 40. By their 70s, many men have levels substantially below their younger peak. Symptoms of low testosterone can include reduced muscle mass and strength, lower bone density, diminished libido, fatigue, mood changes, and reduced spontaneous erections. Many of these symptoms, however, overlap with those of depression, sleep disorders, obesity, and general deconditioning—all of which should be excluded before attributing symptoms to low testosterone. The clinical threshold for considering TRT in men with symptoms is typically a morning total testosterone below 300 ng/dL on two separate measurements. When TRT is appropriate, it can improve energy, muscle mass, bone density, libido, and mood. TRT does not appear to initiate prostate cancer in men with healthy prostates but testosterone "fuels" prostate cancer in men with known or unknown disease. Men with known or suspected prostate cancer should not receive TRT. Men on TRT require regular PSA monitoring, and—critically—TRT suppresses testosterone production, so PSA must be interpreted in this context. Men with low testosterone levels may have artificially low PSA levels before starting TRT. PSA levels may initially rise in response to TRT. Other risks include elevated red blood cell count, increasing clot risk, fluid retention, breast tenderness, and acne. Lifestyle measures—resistance training, adequate sleep, weight management, and stress reduction—can meaningfully raise testosterone levels and alleviate many low-testosterone symptoms and should be tried before TRT is pursued.

Testosterone Therapy Versus Erectile Dysfunction Drugs

Erectile dysfunction (ED) and low testosterone are related but distinct problems that are frequently confused. In men with normal testosterone levels, adding TRT will not meaningfully improve erectile function beyond what ED drugs like sildenafil or tadalafil can achieve on their own. ED in older men is primarily a vascular problem—reduced arterial flow to the erectile tissue—rather than a hormonal one, which is why cardiovascular risk factor management (blood pressure, cholesterol, blood sugar, smoking cessation) is the most important intervention for long-term erectile health. Before attributing ED or "andropause" symptoms to low testosterone, it is worth addressing the modifiable factors that independently improve both: resistance training increases endogenous testosterone and improves blood vessel function; adequate sleep is one of the strongest determinants of morning testosterone levels; weight loss in overweight men reliably raises testosterone. These are not alternatives to treatment—they are the treatment for some men, and should be considered before requesting a testosterone prescription.

Aging and Your Sex Life

Sexual health in older adults is frequently overlooked by clinicians and underreported by patients. Many people remain sexually active and interested in sex well into their 80s and 90s, and the form that intimacy takes may evolve without its importance diminishing. Regular sexual activity is associated with measurable health benefits: improved cardiovascular function, better sleep, reduced psychological distress, and stronger social connection. For women, GSM (described above) is the most common treatable barrier to comfortable sex after menopause, and it responds reliably to local estrogen therapy. Open conversation with both partners and clinicians is essential: most healthcare providers will not raise the topic unless the patient does, and effective treatments exist for the most common problems.

Sexual Health and STI Risk in Older Adults

Sexually transmitted infections (STIs) are rising among older adults—a trend that often surprises patients and clinicians alike. Several factors drive this: women past menopause and men past the age of concern about pregnancy often abandon condom use, reasoning that contraception is no longer needed.

They are correct that contraception is not needed; they are wrong that protection against infection is not. The immune changes of aging (see Chapter 16) also increase susceptibility to STIs. HIV deserves specific mention: the CDC reports that adults 50 and older account for roughly half of Americans living with diagnosed HIV, and older adults with HIV are frequently diagnosed later because fatigue, cognitive changes, and weight loss are attributed to normal aging rather than infection. Rates of syphilis, gonorrhea, and chlamydia among older adults have risen substantially over the past decade. The practical recommendations are the same as at any age: use barrier protection with new or non-exclusive partners, communicate openly about STI status, and discuss appropriate screening with your clinician.

Conclusion

Subclinical hypothyroidism in older adults is a laboratory finding, not a diagnosis that automatically warrants medication. The risks of unnecessary treatment, including atrial fibrillation and bone loss, are real. For women: the 2002 WHI trial was a study of older women, most of whom were well past the window when HRT provides its greatest benefit. For women who initiate HRT within ten years of menopause onset or before age 60, the evidence supports meaningful benefit. The breast cancer risk from combined estrogen-progesterone therapy is real but small, and must be weighed individually against substantial quality-of-life and long-term health benefits. For men: most of what presents as "low testosterone" is the accumulated effect of poor sleep, excess weight, physical deconditioning, and chronic stress—all of which suppress testosterone independently and all of which respond to lifestyle changes more reliably than to a prescription. The frequency with which TRT is prescribed without truly low testosterone levels has made it one of the most overused treatments. For erectile dysfunction, appropriate ED medications address the actual mechanism far more reliably than TRT in men with normal testosterone levels. Finally: sexual health in older adults deserves the same clinical attention as every other domain of health covered in this book. The barriers to comfortable, safe sexual activity—GSM, erectile dysfunction, STI risk from abandoned condom use—are largely treatable. They go undertreated primarily because the topic goes unraised. My suggestion - raise it.

Chapter 13:

Your Eyes and Ears as You Age

VISION AND HEARING ARE among the senses people most fear losing as they age. Age-related changes to both are nearly universal. Many of the conditions covered in this chapter—cataracts, glaucoma, macular degeneration, hearing loss—can be detected early, slowed, or treated effectively when not ignored. The chapter covers the most common age-related conditions of the eyes and ears, the warning signs that require prompt attention, the protective measures that genuinely reduce risk, and the treatments that work. Two overarching principles apply throughout: regular screening catches problems before they cause irreversible harm, and neglecting hearing and vision loss carries costs—social isolation, depression, cognitive decline, and an increased fall risk.

Presbyopia — Age-Related Farsightedness

Beginning in the early-to-mid forties, virtually everyone experiences presbyopia—the progressive loss of the eye's ability to focus on close objects. The cause is mechanical: the crystalline lens gradually stiffens with age, losing the flexibility that allows it to change shape for near focus. Typical symptoms include the need to hold reading material at arm's length, eye strain during sustained close work, and headaches after reading. Unlike most other age-related eye conditions, presbyopia is entirely normal, affects essentially everyone, and has straightforward solutions: reading glasses (over-the-counter or prescription), bifocals, progressive lenses (which blend distance and near correction without a visible line), or contact lens strategies such as monovision. Surgical options that should be discussed with an ophthalmologist, are available for motivated patients who prefer not to wear glasses, though they have trade-offs including loss of depth perception and night vision issues.

Dry Eyes

Dry eyes are among the most common eye complaints in older adults, affecting up to one-third of people over 65. Dry eye results from a combination of reduced tear production and increased tear evaporation. Other symptoms include burning, gritty sensation, redness, and blurred vision that clears with blinking. First-line treatment is frequent use of preservative-free artificial tears (preservatives worsen chronic dry eye with repeated use). Screen time, ceiling fans, air conditioning, and low-humidity environments all worsen dry eyes.

Floaters and Flashes

Floaters are the visible shadow of small clumps of cells and other material within the vitreous—the gel that fills the eye's interior. As the vitreous liquefies and shrinks with age, it eventually separates from the retina. This is extremely common after age 50 and typically causes a sudden increase in floaters and flashes of light. In the vast majority of cases it is benign and the symptoms diminish as the brain adapts. However, in a small percentage of cases—roughly 1 in 10—the separating vitreous tears the retina, which can lead to retinal detachment. Retinal detachment is a sight-threatening emergency. The warning signs are unmistakable and require same-day evaluation: a sudden shower of new floaters, repeated flashing lights, or a curtain, shadow, or dark veil moving across any part of your visual field. Do not wait for a routine appointment. Call an eye doctor or go to an emergency department immediately. Retinal detachment treated promptly almost always preserves vision; untreated, it causes permanent blindness in the affected eye.

Slow Dark Adaptation

Dark adaptation—the process by which the eye adjusts from bright light to darkness—slows with age and is very common by the sixties. A 60-year-old typically requires three to four times longer to adapt to darkness than a 20-year-old, and perceives significantly less detail at equivalent low-light levels. Practical consequences include difficulty entering darkened movie theaters, navigating poorly lit rooms, and—most importantly—driving at night, where oncoming headlights cause prolonged glare recovery that temporarily blinds the driver. Strategies: allow more time when moving from bright to dim environments, increase interior lighting at home (especially on stairs), and take seriously the decision to limit or stop night driving when glare recovery becomes a safety concern. Night driving impairment in older adults is a serious road safety issue.

Cataracts

Cataracts—the gradual clouding of the eye's lens—are among the most prevalent conditions in aging, affecting more than half of Americans by age 80. Most cataracts are the natural result of damage to lens proteins over decades. Accelerating factors include UV exposure, smoking, diabetes, prolonged corticosteroid use (oral or inhaled), and prior eye injury. Symptoms develop gradually: initially increased glare and halos around lights at night, then blurred or hazy vision, fading colors, and eventually significant visual impairment. When cataracts interfere with daily activities—driving, reading, recognizing faces—surgical removal is indicated and highly effective. Cataract surgery is the most commonly performed surgical procedure in the United States. The procedure takes 15 to 30 minutes. Under topical anesthesia, the clouded lens is removed and a permanent lens implant replaces it. Visual recovery is typically rapid; most patients notice improvement within days. Outcomes are excellent: over 95 percent of patients achieve improved vision. The primary preventive measure is UV protection—quality sunglasses that block 100 percent of UVA and UVB rays, worn consistently from early in life. Smoking cessation and blood sugar control in diabetics also reduce cataract progression.

Glaucoma

Glaucoma occurs when fluid in the eye does not drain properly, leading to increased pressure that can harm the optic nerve—the cable connecting your eye to your brain. This increased pressure can be detected by the puff of air during your eye exam. While glaucoma cannot be cured, it can be managed effectively if caught early. That is why regular eye exams are important, even if your vision seems fine. Treatment aims to lower eye pressure through prescription eye drops, oral medications, laser procedures, or conventional surgery.

Age-Related Macular Degeneration (AMD)

AMD is akin to having a worn-out spot in the center of your vision. It occurs when the macula—the small central region of the retina—starts to deteriorate. Patients may notice that when looking at someone's face, they have trouble seeing features clearly but can still see the outline. The dry form of AMD accounts for about 90 percent of cases; it progresses slowly, does not cause blindness, but can make recognizing faces and driving difficult. The more serious wet form involves abnormal blood vessel growth under the retina. These vessels can leak and cause rapid vision loss. Treatment options include eye injections to help stop abnormal blood vessel growth. Patients may also need magnifying glasses and special lighting to cope with vision loss. Early warning signs include straight lines appearing wavy, difficulty reading, and dark or blurry spots in your central vision. If you experience any of these issues, see your eye doctor as soon as possible to maximize your chances of preserving your vision.

Hearing Loss

Aging can also affect hearing, affecting roughly one in three people over 65 and two in three over 75, making it difficult to follow conversations, especially in noisy environments. If you notice hearing difficulties, do not postpone getting a hearing test. Hearing aids can significantly enhance your enjoyment of conversations and media, and they can also reduce feelings of loneliness and isolation—factors linked to health issues like dementia. Hearing loss is one of the most modifiable risk factors for dementia. Research also indicates that individuals who regularly use hearing aids have a 24 percent lower risk of premature death compared to those who do not. Hearing aids have improved dramatically in the past decade and are far less visible and more effective than most patients expect. To protect your hearing, avoid excessive use of medications like NSAIDs or aspirin, use earplugs in loud environments, and keep headphone volumes at moderate levels. Additionally, maintain ear cleanliness without using cotton swabs, which can push earwax deeper or cause injury. The safest way to clean your ears is to only clean what you can see. Earwax has a lot of benefits. If it is decreasing your hearing, have an ear specialist remove the wax.

Tinnitus

Tinnitus is the perception of sound in the head or ears without any external sound present. It is often described as a ringing, buzzing, hissing, whistling, swooshing, or clicking noise. Cognitive behavioral therapy (CBT) adapted for tinnitus is the best-evidenced psychological intervention and reduces tinnitus-related distress and functional impairment in randomized trials. The most common cause of tinnitus is hearing loss. External white noise machines and fans can decrease tinnitus by masking the internal sounds and assisting the brain in ignoring them.

Hearing aids are particularly useful when tinnitus is associated with hearing loss. Avoid silence when tinnitus is bothersome; low background sound is almost always more comfortable than quiet.

Vertigo and Dizziness

Vertigo is a type of dizziness characterized by a false sense of spinning or whirling. The prevalence of vertigo increases significantly with age, making it one of the most common reasons older adults seek medical attention. About half of individuals aged 80 and older may experience vertigo, and women are three times more likely to be affected than men. The most common type of vertigo is called benign paroxysmal positional vertigo (BPPV), which occurs when tiny calcium crystals in the inner ear become dislodged. The Epley Maneuver, which can be found in instructional videos on platforms like YouTube, often resolves BPPV. A single session with this treatment resolves symptoms in approximately 80 percent of patients. If symptoms persist an evaluation by an ear specialist is necessary to rule out other causes of vertigo like infection, or even a stroke. Red flags that demand immediate medical attention rather than home management: vertigo accompanied by sudden headache, double vision, difficulty speaking or swallowing, facial numbness, limb weakness, or inability to walk. These may indicate a stroke and require emergency evaluation (see Chapter 5). In some cases, patients may require specialized physical therapy maneuvers to manage their symptoms effectively.

Conclusion

Age-related changes to eyes and ears are nearly inevitable, but their consequences are far from fixed. Early detection and prompt action determine outcomes. Cataracts are reversible with surgery that ranks among the most successful elective procedures in medicine. Glaucoma is controllable when detected before significant nerve damage occurs—which is why it must be screened for. Wet AMD is treatable with injections that stabilize or improve vision in the majority of patients. Hearing loss is the most significant modifiable dementia risk factor identified, yet remains massively undertreated. BPPV—one of the most disabling forms of vertigo—is curable with a five-minute maneuver. Regular eye and hearing exams are the mechanism by which treatable conditions are caught before they cause permanent harm.

Chapter 14:

The Gut: Your Digestive System

YOUR DIGESTIVE SYSTEM IS essentially a long tube—from mouth to anus—with each section playing a specific role in breaking down food, absorbing nutrients, and eliminating waste. Aging affects every part of this system in predictable ways, most of which can be managed with diet, lifestyle, and when needed, medication. This chapter covers the most common age-related digestive conditions, from dry mouth and heartburn to constipation and colon cancer. Colon cancer is one of the most common cancers in both men and women—and one of the most preventable through regular screening. That screening, and when to get it, is covered at the end of this chapter.

Oral Health

As we age, saliva production tends to decline, leading to dry mouth—which is more than just uncomfortable. Saliva plays an active role in protecting teeth: it rinses away food particles, neutralizes acid, and contains minerals that help repair early tooth decay. Less saliva means more cavities and a higher risk of gum disease. To support oral health, chew sugar-free gum to stimulate saliva flow, drink water, and brush and floss consistently. Regular dental visits matter more than most people realize: gum disease has been linked to heart disease and diabetes, likely because the bacteria involved in gum infections can enter the bloodstream and trigger inflammation elsewhere. Poor oral health can also make chewing difficult, which limits food choices and can quietly contribute to nutritional deficiencies over time.

Gastroesophageal Reflux Disease (GERD) — "Heartburn"

Heartburn—the burning sensation in the chest caused by stomach acid rising into the esophagus—becomes more common with age. The medical term is gastroesophageal reflux disease, or GERD. As we get older, the valve between the esophagus and stomach weakens and the stomach empties more slowly, both of which make reflux more likely. Symptoms include heartburn, chest discomfort, burping, a dry cough, and occasionally hiccups or a sour taste in the mouth.

GERD Treatment

Many GERD cases respond well to simple changes. Losing even a modest amount of weight significantly reduces symptoms. Avoiding fatty foods, spicy foods, chocolate, caffeine, alcohol, and acidic foods helps, as does eating smaller meals. Waiting two to three hours after eating before lying down, and elevating the head of your bed a few inches, prevents acid from pooling at the top of the stomach at night. Loose-fitting clothing reduces abdominal pressure. For quick relief, antacids like Tums or Maalox neutralize acid within minutes. If symptoms are frequent, two classes of medications that reduce acid production more durably: H2 blockers (famotidine, sold as Pepcid) and proton pump inhibitors, or PPIs (omeprazole, sold as Prilosec) are available for use up to 14 days up to three times a year. PPIs are highly effective but should be used at the lowest dose for the shortest time needed—long-term use has been associated with reduced kidney function, increased fracture risk, from a decrease in calcium and magnesium absorption, deficiencies of B12, iron, and magnesium as well as changes to the gut microbiome. I have seen dozens of patients who remain on PPIs for years despite the potential harms. Studies estimate that 25% to 70% on long term PPIs have no clear medical indications for continued use! H2 Blockers are preferred for occassional heartburn and for long term maintenance.

A newer class of acid-suppressing drugs—vonoprazan—works from the first dose and can be taken at any time (traditional PPIs take several days to reach full effect and must be taken before a meal). These are more expensive and generally reserved for cases that do not respond to standard PPIs. As with all medications, discuss the right approach with your doctor.

GERD or Heart Attack?

GERD chest pain and heart attack chest pain can feel similar, and it is important to know the difference—because confusing them can be dangerous. GERD pain tends to burn, worsens when you lie down or bend over, and typically improves within minutes of taking an antacid. Heart-related chest pain is more often described as pressure, tightness, or squeezing, tends to occur with physical activity or stress, and does not improve with antacids. I keep Tums with me and use them as a quick test: if the pain resolves quickly after an antacid, it is almost certainly GERD. If it does not, or if the pain spreads to the left arm, jaw, neck, or back, or comes with shortness of breath, sweating, or nausea, do not wait—call 911 or go to the emergency room immediately. Doctors far prefer to tell you it was indigestion than to learn you waited through a heart attack.

The Gut Microbiome

The gut microbiome is the community of trillions of bacteria, fungi, and other microorganisms that live primarily in the large intestine. Far from being passive passengers, they do essential work: breaking down fiber and complex carbohydrates that our own digestive system cannot process, producing vitamins including K and B12, and sending chemical signals that influence the brain and help regulate the immune system (more on this in Chapter 16). As we age, the microbiome tends to lose diversity—fewer species, less variety. This matters because a diverse microbiome is more resilient: it can recover from disruptions like illness or antibiotics and is better at keeping harmful bacteria in check. Centenarian studies have consistently found that people who reach 100 in good health tend to have unusually diverse microbiomes. The most reliable way to support microbiome diversity is through diet—specifically, eating a wide variety of plant foods rich in fiber, and including fermented foods like yogurt, kefir, kimchi, and sauerkraut.

Diverticulosis and Diverticulitis

Diverticulosis is the presence of small pouches—called

diverticula—that form in weak spots along the wall of the large intestine. It is extremely common with age: more than half of adults over 60 have it, and three out of four do by age 80. Most people never know they have it and never will—diverticulosis causes no symptoms on its own. The problem arises when one of these pouches becomes inflamed or infected, a condition called diverticulitis. Diverticulitis can cause fever, abdominal pain (typically on the lower left side), nausea, and changes in bowel habits, and usually requires antibiotics and sometimes hospitalization. Serious complications like a perforated (ruptured) pouch are uncommon, occurring in less than one in 100 cases of diverticulitis. A high-fiber diet and adequate fluid intake are the primary tools for preventing diverticulosis from progressing and reducing flare-up risk.

Constipation — The Aging Nemesis

Constipation is one of the most common digestive complaints in older adults, affecting roughly one in three people over 65. Aging slows the movement of material through the colon, and many of the medications commonly taken by older adults make it worse—opioid pain medications in particular, but also certain antacids (calcium-based), antihistamines, and some blood pressure medications. If constipation is a persistent problem, it is worth asking your doctor whether any of your current medications could be contributing. The foundations of prevention and management are straightforward: eat more fiber (fruits, vegetables, whole grains, legumes), drink plenty of water, and stay physically active. Exercise stimulates the muscles of the intestinal wall and is one of the most effective natural remedies for sluggish digestion.

Treating Chronic Constipation

When dietary changes alone are not enough, there is a reliable and well-understood treatment ladder. Start by gradually adding soluble fiber—psyllium husk (Metamucil) is the most evidence-backed choice and is better tolerated than insoluble fiber like wheat bran. Increase water intake alongside any fiber increase, aiming for eight to ten cups of fluid daily; without it, fiber can actually worsen constipation by forming a dense mass in the colon. Your colon is naturally most active in the 15 to 45 minutes after a meal, especially breakfast—take advantage of this by setting aside time for the bathroom during that window. A footstool under the feet while sitting on the toilet (the Squatty Potty is the best-known brand) raises the knees above hip level, which straightens the rectal canal and makes passing stool noticeably easier. If these steps are insufficient, polyethylene glycol (MiraLAX) is a safe and effective option for daily, long-term use—it works by drawing water into the stool to keep it soft. Two treatments that are commonly tried but should be avoided for chronic constipation: stimulant laxatives like bisacodyl (Dulcolax) can cause cramping and dependency with regular use, and stool softeners like docusate (Colace) have not been shown to be more effective than placebo for chronic constipation. For people with pelvic floor dysfunction—where the muscles around the rectum do not relax properly during a bowel movement—pelvic floor physical therapy can be highly effective and is an underused resource.

Irritable Bowel Syndrome (IBS)

Irritable bowel syndrome (IBS) is a common condition in which abdominal pain occurs alongside changes in bowel habits—diarrhea, constipation, or both, sometimes alternating. It is not a structural disease but a functional one: the gut is working differently, not damaged. Keeping a food diary to identify personal triggers is often the most useful first step; a dietitian can help. Increasing dietary fiber helps regulate both diarrhea and constipation. Antispasmodic medications like dicyclomine (Bentyl) reduce cramping. Stress is a well-established IBS trigger, and Cognitive Behavioral Therapy (CBT) has good evidence behind it for reducing IBS symptoms by addressing the gut-brain connection. A gastroenterologist can prescribe targeted IBS medications when first-line measures fail, though it is worth knowing upfront that most patients find the greatest benefit from dietary and lifestyle changes rather than medication.

Colon Cancer Prevention

Colon cancer is the third most common cancer in the United States and one of the most preventable, because it typically develops slowly from polyps—small growths on the colon lining—that can be found and removed before they turn cancerous. Colonoscopy is the gold-standard screening test: a flexible camera examines the entire colon, and any polyps found can be removed in the same procedure. Current guidelines recommend starting screening at age 45 for average-risk adults (or earlier with a family history of colon cancer or polyps, which meaningfully raises your risk). Despite being very safe, colonoscopy does involve a day of bowel preparation, sedation, and a small risk of complications including bowel perforation—rare, but worth knowing. For those who prefer to avoid colonoscopy, non-invasive alternatives exist: stool blood tests (FIT test, done annually) and stool DNA tests (Cologuard, done every one to three years) can detect signs of cancer or large polyps. These are good options for people who decline colonoscopy, but they are less comprehensive—any abnormal result requires follow-up with a colonoscopy. For adults between 76 and 85, the decision to continue screening should be individualized based on health status. Screening is generally not recommended past age 85.

Conclusion

The gut responds well to the same principles that benefit the rest of the body: a diet rich in fiber and a variety of plant foods, adequate hydration, and regular physical activity. These habits support a diverse microbiome, keep the colon moving, reduce GERD symptoms, and lower the risk of diverticular disease. If you are on a PPI and have never asked your doctor whether you still need it, ask at your next visit. Up to 70 percent of people on long-term PPIs have no medical indication, which risks kidney damage, fractures, nutrient deficiencies, and microbiome disruption. Also, be up to date on colon cancer screening since it is one of the few cancers that can almost always be prevented entirely when caught at the polyp stage. Do not put off your colonoscopy.

Chapter 15:

Kidney and Urinary Tract Issues

THIS CHAPTER COVERS THE urinary tract conditions that become increasingly common as we age: chronic kidney disease, nighttime urination (nocturia), urinary incontinence, prostate enlargement, prostate cancer screening, kidney stones, erectile dysfunction (ED), pelvic organ prolapse, and urinary tract infections. Most of these conditions are manageable—and some are preventable—with the right information and timely care.

Chronic Kidney Disease (CKD)

The key test for kidney function is the estimated glomerular filtration rate, or eGFR, which measures how efficiently the kidneys are filtering the blood. A normal eGFR is above 60, but it is worth knowing that eGFR naturally declines somewhat with age—for people over 70, an eGFR between 45 and 60 may be considered age-appropriate rather than a sign of disease, particularly if there is little or no protein in the urine. Protein in the urine (proteinuria) is the more worrying finding: it signals that the kidney's filtering barrier is damaged and that the condition is more likely to progress. For most people with CKD stage 3 (eGFR 30 to 60) and low urine protein levels, the real concern is cardiovascular disease, not dialysis. An abnormal eGFR functions much like high blood pressure as a risk factor—it raises the odds of heart disease and should be managed accordingly, with attention to blood pressure, cholesterol, and diet (see earlier chapters). If urine protein levels are consistently elevated, medications called ACE inhibitors, ARBs (see Chapter 3), or SGLT2 inhibitors (see Chapter 4) can reduce protein leakage, slow kidney function decline, and lower cardiovascular risk. One important point about dialysis: research suggests that in the U.S. and other developed countries, many patients begin dialysis earlier than necessary—often at eGFR values above 10. International studies have shown that starting dialysis at eGFR levels of 5 to 10 or lower may produce equal or better patient survival and quality of life. If you have CKD and want to go deeper, I cover all of these issues in my book "Learn the Facts About Kidney Disease" and on the YouTube channel (Dadvice TV).

Nocturia — Nighttime Urination

Nocturia—waking up at night to urinate—is one of the most common and underappreciated disruptors of sleep for older adults. As we age, the body produces less of the hormone that signals the kidneys to reduce urine output overnight. The bladder loses elasticity and may become overactive and this may trigger a full bladder sensation. In people with heart failure or leg swelling, fluid that accumulates during the day gets reabsorbed when lying down and routed to the bladder at night. Practical steps to reduce nocturia: limit fluids in the two to three hours before bed, and cut back on caffeine and alcohol in the afternoon and evening, as both increase urine production. Elevating the legs for an hour before bedtime can help people with leg swelling pass fluid earlier in the evening rather than overnight.

Urinary Incontinence

Urinary incontinence—leaking urine—is common in older adults but is not an inevitable part of aging, and many people are too embarrassed to mention it to their doctor. There are several types, each with different causes. Stress incontinence is leakage triggered by physical pressure on the bladder—coughing, sneezing, laughing, or lifting—most often in women whose pelvic floor muscles have weakened after childbirth. Overflow incontinence occurs when the bladder never fully empties and eventually leaks; in men, an enlarged prostate is the most common cause. Urge incontinence is a sudden, intense need to urinate that can be difficult to defer; it may signal a bladder infection but is also common with an overactive bladder. Knowing which type you have matters because treatments differ and should be discussed with your urologist and gynecologist.

Treatment of Urinary Incontinence

For stress incontinence (leaking urine when the bladder is put under pressure), pelvic floor exercises—Kegels—are the first-line treatment and are effective for both women and men. For women, a pessary—a small, flexible silicone device inserted into the vagina to support the pelvic floor—can provide meaningful relief without medication or surgery. Bladder training (gradually lengthening the intervals between urination) helps with urge incontinence. Medications are available for both overactive bladder and BPH-related symptoms (described in the BPH section below). If you are experiencing incontinence, bring it up with your doctor: it is treatable, and suffering in silence is unnecessary.

The PSA Test

The PSA (prostate-specific antigen) test measures a protein produced by the prostate gland. High levels can indicate prostate cancer, but they are far more commonly caused by an enlarged prostate or prostate inflammation. Most men with an elevated PSA do not have prostate cancer, but the result triggers biopsies, which can lead to diagnosing slow-growing cancers that would never have caused symptoms or shortened a man's life—followed by surgery or radiation that carry real risks of incontinence and erectile dysfunction. Research estimates that for every prostate cancer death potentially prevented by aggressive screening and treatment, roughly 26 men are overdiagnosed and treated unnecessarily. This has led some experts to call routine PSA screening a public health problem. The U.S. Preventive Services Task Force recommends that men aged 55 to 69 have an informed conversation with their doctor about the benefits and harms of PSA screening, and advises against routine screening for men 70 and older where the likelihood of harm as a result of the test is much higher than the likelihood that the test might save your life. The takeaway: an elevated PSA is not an automatic mandate for aggressive action. Talk to your doctor about what it means for you specifically.

Benign Prostatic Hyperplasia (BPH)

Benign prostatic hyperplasia—BPH, or prostate enlargement—is almost universal in older men: by age 80, nine out of ten have it. It causes symptoms because the enlarged gland compresses the urethra, the tube that carries urine out of the body. Typical symptoms include a weak or slow urine stream, difficulty starting urination, dribbling at the end, frequent urination, and waking at night to urinate. If symptoms are mild, simple measures help: reduce fluid intake in the evening, limit caffeine and alcohol, and practice double voiding—after urinating, wait a moment and try again to empty the bladder more completely. When symptoms are more bothersome, medications are the usual next step. Alpha-blockers like tamsulosin (Flomax) or doxazosin (Cardura) relax the muscles around the prostate and bladder neck, improving flow often within days. Finasteride (Proscar) works differently, gradually shrinking the prostate over six to twelve months. The two classes are often combined. If medications are not enough, minimally invasive procedures offer relief without major surgery. One example is Rezum, which uses targeted steam to reduce prostate tissue; there are several others worth discussing with your urologist.

Prostate Cancer

Prostate cancer is the most commonly diagnosed cancer in men, but most men who have it do not die from it—they die of something else first. The cancer often grows so slowly that it never causes symptoms or threatens life. This is the context in which PSA numbers matter. BPH alone typically raises PSA to about 2 to 7 ng/mL. PSA levels between 4 and 10 carry roughly a 25 percent chance of cancer being present; above 10, the risk rises above 50 percent. But a high PSA does not mean aggressive treatment is automatically needed. For men with low-to-intermediate risk prostate cancer, active surveillance—regular PSA checks, repeat biopsies if needed, and MRI monitoring—has become the preferred approach at many centers, avoiding the side effects of treatment unless the cancer shows signs of progression. When a biopsy is needed, many urologists now use an MRI-guided approach, which is more accurate and more comfortable than the traditional method. Black men face roughly twice the risk of prostate cancer and tend to be diagnosed at younger ages—earlier and more attentive screening is warranted for this group.

Kidney Stones

Kidney stones become more common with age, partly because older adults tend to drink less and partly because bones release more calcium as they thin—and that calcium can end up in the urine. The most common stones are calcium oxalate. The most effective prevention is staying well hydrated: aim for at least two liters (roughly two quarts) of water daily. Dietary calcium—from food rather than supplements—actually helps prevent calcium oxalate stones by binding oxalate in the gut before it can be absorbed. When eating high-oxalate foods like spinach, beets, nuts, or chocolate, pair them with a dairy product or other calcium source. High-salt diets increase calcium excretion in the urine, raising stone risk, so cutting back on sodium helps. Citrus drinks like lemonade increase urinary citrate, which inhibits stone formation—a useful addition for individuals with a history of kidney stones.

How Much Water Should You Drink?

The "eight glasses a day" rule has no scientific basis—for most healthy people, drinking when thirsty is sufficient. The body regulates hydration well. That said, thirst becomes a less reliable signal with age, and there are specific situations where drinking more deliberately matters: a history of kidney stones, high heat or heavy sweating, recurrent UTIs, and chronic constipation. In hot weather or during strenuous activity, hydrate proactively rather than waiting for thirst.

Bottled Water and Additives

For most people, tap water is perfectly adequate. If you exercise hard or sweat heavily, a sports drink can help replace electrolytes—sodium and potassium in particular. Beyond that, the premium bottled water market is largely marketing. Products claiming benefits from added vitamins, hydrogen, or alkalinity have little or no scientific support for those claims. Many also contain sugar or artificial sweeteners, making them nutritionally similar to a soft drink. Save your money.

Erectile Dysfunction

Erectile dysfunction (ED) becomes more common with age and is more often a vascular problem than a hormonal one—the same processes that narrow coronary arteries (see Chapter

3) reduce blood flow to the penis. For men in their 30s to 60s, difficulty with getting or maintaining an erection may be an indicator that you are at risk of a heart attack. Discuss this with your doctor.

ED medications—sildenafil (Viagra), tadalafil (Cialis), and vardenafil (Levitra)—are safe and effective for most men and have become much more affordable. One critical safety warning: these medications must never be combined with nitrate drugs such as nitroglycerin or isosorbide dinitrate, used for chest pain. The combination can cause a sudden, dangerous drop in blood pressure. If you take nitrates, discuss this with your doctor before considering ED medication. Lifestyle factors that reduce ED risk and can improve existing ED include not smoking, limiting alcohol, maintaining a healthy weight, and regular cardiovascular exercise. Low testosterone can contribute to ED in some men (see Chapter 12).

Pelvic Organ Prolapse

Pelvic organ prolapse occurs when the muscles and ligaments supporting the pelvic organs—bladder, uterus, or rectum—weaken, allowing one or more organs to press into or protrude through the vaginal wall. Symptoms can include pressure or a feeling of heaviness in the pelvis, a visible or palpable bulge, urinary urgency, incontinence, constipation, and other bowel difficulties. It is extremely common—more than half of women over 80 have some degree of prolapse, though many have mild cases that cause no symptoms and need no treatment. Pelvic floor exercises (Kegels) can improve mild cases. A pessary—a removable silicone device fitted by a clinician—provides support without surgery and works well for many women. Surgery is reserved for cases where symptoms significantly impair quality of life and conservative management has not helped.

Urinary Tract Infections (UTIs)

UTIs are more frequent in older adults for different reasons in men and women. In women, the drop in estrogen after menopause thins the tissues of the urethra and vagina, making them more vulnerable to bacterial invasion. In men, an enlarged prostate that prevents the bladder from fully emptying creates stagnant urine where bacteria can grow. Prevention strategies: stay well hydrated (dilute urine flushes bacteria from the urinary tract), urinate regularly and make sure the bladder empties fully, and for women, wipe front to back and urinate after sexual activity. Postmenopausal women with recurrent UTIs should ask their doctor about vaginal estrogen—a local estrogen cream or suppository that is highly effective at reducing UTI recurrence and has minimal absorption into the bloodstream.

Conclusion

One thread that runs through this chapter, is the cost of not speaking up. Urinary incontinence affects one in three older women and is mentioned to a physician by fewer than half of them. Erectile dysfunction affects the majority of men over 70 and many of these men do not raise the issue with their provider. Pelvic organ prolapse causes suffering for years in a many older women, before they bring the issue up. Effective treatments exist for all of these conditions. Suffering in silence is unnecessary.

Hydration, a low-sodium diet, blood pressure control, blood sugar management, and regular physical activity can help protect kidney and urinary function. An elevated PSA should be managed conservatively for most men. Before agreeing to a biopsy or a surgical procedure discuss all the options with your urologist. CKD at stage 3 with low urine protein is often a cardiovascular risk factor more than a kidney disease that should be managed accordingly (see Chapters 1-4). If you have elevated urine protein as well as an abnormal kidney number (eGFR) there are many new treatments that can decrease urine protein and slow the decline of kidney function. Check out my DadviceTV talks and my kidney book "Learn the Facts About Kidney Disease" to learn more.

Chapter 16:

The Immune System and Aging

THE IMMUNE SYSTEM IS the body's defense network. Two of its most important cell types are T cells, which hunt and destroy infected or cancerous cells, and B cells, which produce antibodies—proteins that tag foreign invaders for destruction. Both weaken with age. T cells are made in the thymus gland, which begins shrinking after puberty and is largely replaced by fat by the time we reach our sixties. With fewer fresh T cells available, the immune system struggles to respond effectively to threats it has not encountered before. B cells become less efficient at producing antibodies, which is why older adults tend to get sicker from infections like flu and pneumonia, take longer to recover, and do not always mount as strong a response to vaccines. A less vigilant immune system also does a less thorough job of detecting and destroying abnormal cells before they become cancer—one reason cancer risk rises with age.

"Inflammaging": Heightened Inflammation Levels

Alongside the weakening of active immune defenses, aging brings a paradoxical increase in background inflammation. Researchers call this "inflammaging": a persistent, low-grade inflammatory state that increases with aging, as the body accumulates damaged cells and loses some of its ability to clear cellular debris. Unlike the acute inflammation that flares during an infection and then resolves, inflammaging smolders quietly in the background—and that chronic slow burn can affect many of the common diseases of aging. Heart disease, type 2 diabetes, Alzheimer's dementia, and certain cancers all have inflammation as a contributing factor. The same immune dysregulation can also cause the immune system to turn against the body's own tissues, which is why autoimmune conditions like rheumatoid arthritis and lupus become more common with age. Inflammaging is not inevitable, and lifestyle choices can have a meaningful impact.

"Inflammaging" and Your Gut Microbiome

The gut microbiome plays a significant and underappreciated role in driving or reducing inflammaging. After about age 70, the diversity of bacterial species in the gut tends to decline. A less diverse microbiome produces less of the short-chain fatty acids (SCFAs) that healthy gut bacteria generate when they break down fiber. SCFAs do important work: they nourish the cells lining the intestinal wall, strengthen the gut barrier, and actively suppress inflammation throughout the body. When SCFA production falls, the gut wall becomes more permeable—sometimes called "leaky gut"—allowing bacterial fragments to slip into the bloodstream and trigger systemic inflammatory responses. This microbiome-driven inflammation is linked to frailty—age-related decline that includes unintentional weight loss, muscle weakness, slow walking speed, and exhaustion—and may also connect to Alzheimer's and other chronic diseases.

The good news is that the microbiome responds to diet, and the changes needed to improve it are straightforward.

What Helps and Hurts Your Gut Microbiome

The single most important thing you can do for your gut microbiome is eat a wide variety of plants. Different bacterial species thrive on different types of fiber, so variety—vegetables, fruits, legumes, whole grains, nuts, seeds, and herbs—feeds a broader range of species and maintains diversity. Adding at least one serving of fermented food daily—yogurt, kefir, kimchi, sauerkraut, or miso—provides live bacteria that support a healthy microbiome. Antibiotics can kill beneficial bacteria along with harmful ones and should only be used when necessary; they do nothing for viral infections. Proton pump inhibitors (see chapter 14) PPI such as omeprazole/Prilosec and lansoprazole/Prevacid), used long-term, reduce stomach acid in ways that allow bacteria to colonize parts of the gut where they do not belong. Emulsifiers in ultra-processed foods—including many products marketed as "health bars"—thin the protective mucus layer of the intestinal wall. Artificial sweeteners including aspartame and saccharin alter the microbiome in ways that can impair blood sugar regulation. High alcohol intake reduces anti-inflammatory bacterial species. Chronic stress disrupts the gut-brain axis in ways that increase gut permeability. Low fiber intake is perhaps the most common and most correctable driver of microbiome decline (see Chapter 2).

How to Enhance Immune Function

Several lifestyle factors have a direct and meaningful impact on immune function and inflammation levels. Exercise is arguably the most potent anti-inflammatory tool available without a prescription. It reduces visceral fat—the "belly fat" that sits around the abdominal organs and acts as an active source of inflammatory signals—and directly modulates immune cell activity. Even moderate regular exercise consistently reduces markers of inflammation. Sleep is equally important: during sleep the immune system consolidates immune memory, clears inflammatory debris, and resets inflammatory signaling. Chronic poor sleep raises inflammatory markers and weakens immune responses to vaccines. Aim for seven to nine hours. Chronic stress elevates cortisol, which suppresses immune function and promotes inflammation over time; stress management practices—whether meditation, yoga, deep breathing, time in nature, or connection with people you care about—have measurable anti-inflammatory effects. Staying well hydrated supports the production of lymph (which circulates immune cells), as well as saliva, tears, and mucus—the body's first-line physical barriers against bacteria and viruses.

Vaccinations Enhance Immune Function

For aging adults with a weakening immune system, vaccines are especially valuable. They work by training the immune system to recognize a pathogen in advance, so that if the real infection arrives, the response is faster and stronger than a weakened aging immune system could mount from scratch. Preventing severe infections also matters beyond the infection itself: a serious bout of flu or pneumonia can trigger inflammatory spikes that increase the short-term risk of heart attack and stroke, and contribute to longer-term cognitive decline. An annual high-dose or adjuvanted flu vaccine is specifically formulated for adults 65 and older, as standard doses produce weaker responses, and is recommended every fall. The shingles vaccine (Shingrix) requires two doses and is recommended for everyone 50 and older; research suggests it is also associated with reduced dementia risk, likely by preventing the significant inflammatory event that shingles causes. A pneumococcal vaccine protects against bacterial pneumonia and is recommended for adults 50 and older (ask your doctor when and which formulation you should get). An RSV vaccine is recommended for adults 75 and older, or 60 and older with certain risk factors. Annual COVID vaccination is also recommended. If you are unsure which vaccines you have had or are due for, ask your pharmacist or primary care provider to review your vaccination history.

Conclusion

As we age the immune system's active defenses weaken while background inflammation increases. Both trends raise the risk of infection, cancer, chronic disease, and cognitive decline. The encouraging reality is that both are responsive to lifestyle: the same habits that protect the heart and brain—regular exercise, a varied plant-rich diet, adequate sleep, stress management, and staying hydrated—also reduce inflammaging and support immune function. Regular exercise is the most potent anti-inflammatory tool available - it reduces visceral fat, modulates immune cell activity, and consistently lowers inflammatory markers. A healthy gut microbiome is a key part of this picture, and it is shaped more by what you eat than by any supplement (see Chapter 19). A varied, plant-rich diet with adequate fiber and fermented foods is the most direct intervention available for the gut microbiome. A low fiber high ultra-processed food diet, unnecessary antibiotics and long-term PPIs all drive up inflammation that can accelerate aging. Adequate sleep is necessary for the immune system to do its maintenance work. Chronic stress, left unmanaged, continuously elevates cortisol in ways that suppress immune function and promote inflammation. A serious bout of flu or pneumonia in an older adult does not simply resolve — it can trigger inflammatory spikes that increase the short-term risk of heart attack and stroke and cognitive decline. Staying current on recommended vaccines is one of the most direct ways to compensate for immune decline and protect against the consequences of severe infections.

Chapter 17:

Your Breathing Apparatus

YOUR LUNGS AND AIRWAYS are designed to last a lifetime, but aging affects them in ways that matter for everyday health. This chapter covers the respiratory conditions that become more common with age: the gradual changes to airways and lung capacity, chronic cough, sleep apnea, and the consequences of smoking. Vaccinations that protect against respiratory infections are covered in Chapter 16.

Age and Our Airways

With age, the lungs gradually lose some of their natural elasticity—the ability to expand fully and spring back. The breathing muscles weaken, and the tiny hairlike structures lining the airways (cilia), which sweep mucus and debris upward and out, become less efficient. The practical result is a decline in lung capacity, slower clearance of mucus after infections, and a longer recovery from respiratory illness. For most healthy non-smokers these changes are gradual and manageable.

Chronic Cough and Allergy Symptoms

A cough that lingers for weeks after a respiratory infection is common in older adults. As cilia become less efficient with age, the airways rely more on coughing to clear mucus. Staying well hydrated is the simplest first step—it keeps mucus thinner and easier to move. A humidifier helps in dry indoor environments, particularly in winter. If the cough is producing mucus, an expectorant like guaifenesin (Mucinex) helps loosen it. A cough suppressant like dextromethorphan suits a dry, non-productive cough—using a cough suppressant when there is mucus to clear is counterproductive. Allergies and post-nasal drip are another common cause of persistent cough. For daytime allergy symptoms, a non-sedating antihistamine like cetirizine (Zyrtec) or loratadine (Claritin) works well. For nighttime symptoms, diphenhydramine (Benadryl, 25 mg) can help, but use it cautiously in older adults—it can cause confusion, urinary retention, and next-day grogginess. Nasal corticosteroid sprays like fluticasone (Flonase) are highly effective for allergic nasal symptoms and post-nasal drip and are safe for regular use. A post-infection cough lasting more than a few weeks, producing blood, or accompanied by fever, shortness of breath, or unexplained weight loss should be evaluated by your health care provider.

Sleep Apnea

Sleep apnea affects an estimated 30 million Americans, and the true number is likely higher because many cases go undiagnosed. It becomes more common with age and weight gain, and is more prevalent in men. The most common form, obstructive sleep apnea (OSA), occurs when the soft tissues at the back of the throat collapse during sleep, repeatedly blocking the airway. Each blockage briefly rouses the brain just enough to restore breathing, fragmenting sleep without the person realizing it. Central sleep apnea is less common and involves the brain failing to send the breathing signal rather than a physical obstruction. Typical symptoms include loud snoring, witnessed episodes of stopped breathing, gasping or choking awake, dry mouth or sore throat in the morning, and—most commonly—excessive daytime sleepiness despite adequate time in bed. Untreated OSA raises the risk of high blood pressure, heart attack, stroke, and type 2 diabetes, and meaningfully impairs memory, concentration, and driving safety. The standard treatment is CPAP (continuous positive airway pressure)—a bedside machine that delivers a gentle stream of pressurized air through a mask to keep the airway open all night. Consistent CPAP use improves daytime energy, memory, and mood, and reduces cardiovascular risk. The challenge is adherence: about half of people prescribed CPAP do not maintain it long-term. Mask discomfort and the sensation of pressurized air are the most common barriers, but most can be resolved with the right mask fit, pressure adjustments, or a heated humidifier attachment—a sleep specialist or respiratory therapist can help. For those who genuinely cannot tolerate CPAP, alternatives include dental appliances that reposition the jaw, positional therapy for mild OSA, and in selected cases, surgical options. If you snore heavily or wake unrefreshed despite adequate sleep, ask your doctor about a sleep study.

Smoking — The Leading Cause of Preventable Death and Disease

Smoking is the leading cause of preventable death and disease in the United States. Its respiratory consequences alone are severe: it is the primary cause of chronic obstructive pulmonary disease (COPD)—which includes chronic bronchitis and emphysema—and the risk rises with every additional year and every additional pack. Beyond the lungs, smoking causes cancers of the mouth, throat, esophagus, stomach, pancreas, kidney, bladder, and cervix, weakens the immune system, and increases the risk of heart disease and stroke discussed in Chapters 3 and 4. The body begins repairing itself within hours of the last cigarette. Quitting at any age brings meaningful benefits: less coughing and breathlessness, improved sense of taste and smell, better lung function, and significantly lower risk of heart attack, stroke, and cancer. Quitting also protects family members—particularly children—from the well-documented harms of secondhand smoke, and cessation treatment may be covered by your health insurance. Nicotine replacement therapy—patches, gum, lozenges, or inhalers—combined with prescription medication (varenicline/Chantix or bupropion/Wellbutrin) significantly improves quit rates compared to willpower alone. If you smoke, quitting is the single highest-impact health action you can take.

Conclusion

The respiratory system ages gradually and—for non-smokers—relatively gently. Regular aerobic exercise is the most effective way to maintain lung capacity and respiratory fitness as the airways age. The two conditions in this chapter that cause the most harm are sleep apnea, which is underdiagnosed and highly treatable, and smoking, which is the most destructive thing a person can do to their lungs and cardiovascular system and the most rewarding thing to stop. If you snore heavily, wake unrefreshed, or have been told you stop breathing during sleep ask your provider about a sleep study. Sleep apnea is associated with elevated blood pressure, increased cardiovascular risk, impaired memory, concentration, and driving safety, and persistent daytime fatigue. If you smoke, no other single action available to you will do as much for your health as stopping. Managing chronic cough, with the right treatment can prevent weeks of unnecessary discomfort. A cough that persists beyond three or four weeks, produces blood, or comes with fever, weight loss, or shortness of breath warrants an evaluation by your medical provider.

SECTION THREE:

The mind, experimental therapy, and the future of medicine

THIS SECTION TURNS TO the inner life of aging -Chapter 18 examines the mental health challenges that accompany growing older—depression, suicide risk, loneliness, and the habits that build resilience and well-being. Chapter 19 reviews experimental longevity interventions, weighing the evidence for and against. Chapter 20 looks at how artificial intelligence is beginning to reshape medicine and what that may mean for how we age.

Chapter 18:

The Mind Matters: Navigating Mental Health in Aging

MENTAL HEALTH AND PHYSICAL health are not separate systems—they are deeply intertwined. Depression worsens outcomes in heart disease, diabetes, and dementia. Chronic pain and illness drive depression. Loneliness raises the risk of early death as much as smoking. This chapter examines the mental health challenges as we age, and more importantly, what actually helps.

Depression

Depression in older adults often goes unrecognized—both by the people experiencing it and by their doctors. The triggers are real and often multiple: retirement can strip away structure, identity, and daily purpose all at once; the cumulative losses of spouses, close friends, and contemporaries are a form of grief that accumulates quietly over years; chronic illness—Parkinson's, heart disease, diabetes—adds physical suffering and loss of independence; and transitions like giving up driving or moving into assisted living can feel like surrendering control over one's own life. Biology compounds these pressures. Reduced blood flow to the brain—from the vascular disease discussed in Chapters 4 and 5—can directly damage the brain networks that regulate mood. The result is sometimes called vascular depression, and it is more common than many people realize. One reason depression goes undetected is that when compared to younger people who are likely to report sadness directly, for older adults depression often surfaces as mental fog (sometimes mistaken for early dementia), increased irritability, withdrawal from activities previously enjoyed and unexplained physical symptoms like persistent headaches or digestive problems. Depression is treatable at any age—but only if it is recognized. If these patterns sound familiar, a conversation with a doctor or mental health professional is the right next step.

Suicide

Older men have among the highest suicide rates of any demographic group, a fact that rarely receives the public attention it warrants. Suicide attempts in this group are more lethal as a result of their access to firearms and their greater likelihood of living alone, with fewer opportunities for intervention. Untreated pain and sleep disorders are significant and underappreciated contributors to suicide risk; addressing them directly can make a meaningful difference. For those at elevated risk, securing or removing access to firearms and reviewing medications to prevent dangerous stockpiling are practical protective steps that family members and clinicians can take. Isolation is among the most powerful drivers of suicide. Simple, structured interventions—regular phone check-ins, befriending programs, involvement in community activities—have been shown to reduce distress and create the kind of informal safety net where changes in behavior get noticed. Connections across generations matter too: adults who mentor, tutor, or engage with younger people consistently report a stronger sense of purpose and are less likely to feel like a burden. If you are concerned about yourself or someone you know, the 988 Suicide and Crisis Lifeline is available in Canada and the U.S. by call or text around the clock. If you are outside the U.S. and Canada, look up the International Association for Suicide Prevention (IASP) to find crisis services in your area.

Cognitive Health and Mental Health

The brain processes that drive cognitive decline and depression in aging adults overlap considerably—which is why treating one often helps the other. Reduced blood flow from atherosclerosis damages mood-regulating circuits just as it damages memory circuits (see Chapters 4–6). This means that the habits that protect the brain—controlling blood pressure, staying active, not smoking—also protect mental health. "Cognitive reserve"—the brain's ability to adapt and compensate as it ages—is built over a lifetime through education, intellectually demanding work, and sustained social engagement. People who have maintained these habits tend to show greater resilience against both cognitive and emotional setbacks in later life. This does not mean that cognitive decline is inevitable for those with less cognitive reserve. It means that staying mentally and socially active is genuinely protective for everyone.

Lifestyle Factors

The lifestyle factors with the strongest evidence for promoting mental health are largely the same as the ones that protect physical health. Regular physical exercise is the single most evidence-backed intervention for depression: it reduces brain inflammation, raises mood, and is as effective as antidepressants for mild to moderate depression in multiple trials. Social connection is equally important and is covered in the Loneliness section below. A Mediterranean-style diet—rich in vegetables, fish, olive oil, legumes, and whole grains—is associated with lower rates of depression, likely through its anti-inflammatory effects on the brain. Mindfulness practices including yoga, tai chi, and simple breathing exercises reduce anxiety and improve emotional regulation; even ten minutes of daily practice can have beneficial effects. Sleep disruption both causes and worsens depression. Protecting sleep quality is one of the most important mental health practices available (see Chapter 6).

Cultivating Resilience

Resilience—the ability to absorb setbacks and adapt—is sometimes treated as a fixed personality trait, but research suggests it functions more like a skill that can be built and strengthened. As you age, you have a genuine advantage: decades of navigating difficulty create a deep, often underappreciated reservoir of coping experience. The "I have been through hard things before" perspective is not denial—it is an accurate and evidence-based reason for confidence. Maintaining a sense of agency over one's own life is central to resilience. This includes involvement in medical and lifestyle decisions rather than having them made by others, learning assistive technologies that preserve independence (hearing aids, mobility aids, home safety modifications—see Chapters 10 and 13), and seeking out peer relationships with others navigating similar transitions. Those shared experiences validate what can otherwise feel like uniquely personal losses. The common thread is connection—with other people, with purpose, with one's own sense of competence. Isolation is the enemy of resilience.

The Loneliness Epidemic

Loneliness has been formally recognized as a public health crisis by the U.S. Surgeon General and the World Health Organization—and the health data behind that designation is striking. Chronic loneliness carries a mortality risk comparable to smoking 15 cigarettes a day. It is associated with a 29 percent higher risk of heart disease, a 32 percent higher risk of stroke, and significantly accelerated cognitive decline. Some researchers now argue that social connection should be treated as a vital sign, measured and addressed as routinely as blood pressure. The transitions of later life create particular vulnerability: losing a spouse, retiring, losing the ability to drive, or moving to a new location can change a person's social world quickly. Prevention and repair require deliberate effort. Staying involved in community activities, clubs, religious or spiritual communities, or volunteer work provides regular structured contact. Maintaining relationships with family and friends through whatever means are accessible—in person, by phone, by video, even by text—matters more than the medium. Having a regular exercise partner combines two of the most important protective factors: physical activity and social connection.

Gratitude

Gratitude practices have a strong evidence base. Regularly directing attention toward what is going well—even small things—trains the brain's pattern-recognition systems to notice positive experiences more readily and not to dwell on losses. Keeping a daily gratitude journal, listing three specific things that went well or that you appreciated, has been shown in controlled studies to increase positive affect, reduce depressive symptoms, and improve sleep. The practice is simple, costs nothing, and requires no particular belief system—just a few minutes of daily reflection.

Looking on the Bright Side: Optimism

Optimism—the general expectation that things will work out—predicts longevity with surprising consistency. Studies from Harvard and Boston University following people over decades have found that those with higher optimism scores are more likely to reach age 85 compared to less optimistic peers. The mechanisms are partly behavioral: optimists tend to engage in healthier habits, adhere better to medical recommendations, and maintain stronger social ties. But there also appear to be direct physiological effects: optimists show lower markers of chronic inflammation and lower rates of heart disease and stroke even after controlling for healthy behaviors. Importantly, optimism is not a fixed disposition. Cognitive reframing—deliberately practicing the habit of looking for what is working rather than what is not—can shift your outlook over time. This is not wishful thinking; it is a trainable mental habit with measurable health benefits.

Conclusion

Mental health deserves the same attention and proactive care as physical health—and the two are less separable than most people assume. Depression, loneliness, and loss of purpose are not inevitable features of aging. Recognizing these problems early and responding appropriately can make a real difference. The tools with the strongest evidence are not complicated: regular exercise, social engagement, adequate sleep, a good diet, and deliberate attention to gratitude and purpose. Resilience, gratitude, and optimism are not just characteristics that some people are fortunate enough to be born with, they are also practices. People who deliberately direct attention toward what is working rather than what is lost, who maintain expectations that things will improve, and who engage with difficulty as something to be navigated rather than endured, live longer, recover faster from illness, and report better quality of life. Exercise works as well as antidepressants for mild to moderate depression. The loneliness epidemic deserves particular emphasis because it is both the most prevalent mental health challenge in older adults and the most amenable to intervention.

Chapter 19:

Experimental Aging Remedies

THE ANTI-AGING SUPPLEMENT AND longevity clinic market exceeds $75 billion a year and is growing rapidly. It is also largely unregulated and heavily marketed to exactly the people most likely to be looking for solutions—adults who are watching their health change and want to do something about it. This chapter reviews the most talked-about experimental interventions: what the science actually shows, what the risks are, and where the genuine promise lies. The guiding principle throughout is the oldest one in medicine: first, do no harm. An important baseline for evaluating all of these claims: over 100 methods have been found to extend lifespan in mice, but only about 3 in 100 drugs that work in rodents prove effective in humans. Many people report feeling better on experimental therapies—but separating a genuine drug effect from the placebo effect, or from lifestyle improvements that often accompany joining a wellness program, is very difficult without a properly designed study where one group receives the treatment, a second similar group receives a placebo, and neither group knows which they are getting—a randomized controlled trial (RCT).

Aging at the Molecular Level (see Chapter 8)

Longevity clinics and supplement companies often invoke the molecular biology of aging to justify their products. The science is real, even if the products built on top of it often are not. As we age, the cellular machinery that repairs DNA becomes less efficient, and errors accumulate—mutations, chromosomal breaks, and copying mistakes that may underlie the rising cancer risk that comes with age. Separately, the epigenetic switches that control which genes are active and which are silent are also affected. Aging cells also lose the ability to fold proteins correctly, and misfolded proteins can contribute to disease. Whether any available supplement or clinic procedure meaningfully corrects these genetic issues for patients is far from established.

Telomeres

Every chromosome in your cells is capped at both ends by telomeres—repetitive stretches of DNA that work like the plastic tips on shoelaces, preventing the chromosome from fraying. Each time a cell divides, the telomere gets slightly shorter. When it becomes too short, the cell can no longer divide—it enters a state called senescence (more on this below) or dies. Short telomeres are associated with accelerated aging, atherosclerosis, type 2 diabetes, weakened immune function, and neurodegenerative diseases including Alzheimer's and Parkinson's.

Lifestyle Choices and Telomeres

The good news about telomeres is that lifestyle choices genuinely influence their rate of shortening. A Mediterranean diet, regular physical activity, adequate sleep, and stress management are all associated with longer telomeres in population studies. Smoking and heavy alcohol use accelerate shortening. This is one of the clearest molecular-level arguments for the lifestyle habits recommended throughout this book.

Telomere Research

In theory, restoring telomere length could rejuvenate aging cells—and this is an active area of legitimate research, with potential applications in diseases driven by cell loss, including certain forms of macular degeneration (Chapter 13) and sarcopenia (Chapter 10). The complication is that longer telomeres are also a feature of cancer cells. Cancer cells stay immortal by using an enzyme called telomerase to maintain their telomeres indefinitely—which is why telomerase inhibitors are actually being explored as cancer treatments. Any therapy designed to lengthen telomeres in healthy cells has to consider this risk carefully. No safe, proven telomere-lengthening therapy for humans currently exists.

Stem Cells

Stem cells are the body's master cells—capable of becoming almost any specialized cell type the body needs, from blood cells to nerve cells to muscle fibers. They are the foundation of tissue repair throughout life. As we age, the number and function of stem cells decline, which is one reason healing slows and tissues lose their resilience. Stem cell research is one of the most genuinely promising areas of longevity science—but the gap between legitimate research and the unregulated clinic market is enormous and important to understand.

Current Uses of Stem Cells

Established stem cell therapies exist and are medically well-supported. Bone marrow transplantation—in which a patient's diseased marrow is destroyed with high-dose radiation and replaced with donor stem cells that rebuild a healthy blood system—has been used successfully in patients with blood cancers and bone marrow disorders. Stem cells have also been used in corneal transplantation to restore vision. These are evidence-based, hospital-based procedures with established safety profiles.

Stem Cell Research

The frontier of stem cell research is focused on two areas with significant long-term promise. The first is reprogramming: taking mature cells and reverting them to an immature stem-cell-like state, then using them to replace damaged tissue in the same patient—avoiding the rejection risk that comes with organ tissue from a donor. The second is combining stem cell therapy with gene editing tools like CRISPR (see Chapter 8) to correct genetic defects before transplanting cells back into the body. Researchers have also created "diseases in a dish"—organ-like structures grown from a patient's own stem cells that reproduce a patient's disease—allowing thousands of potential drugs to be tested in a lab without exposing patients to risk. These are legitimate and exciting areas of research, not yet available as treatments outside of clinical trials.

Unregulated Stem Cell Clinics

Unregulated stem cell clinics are a serious and ongoing patient safety problem. The FDA has documented numerous cases of patients harmed by procedures at these clinics, including infections from contaminated products, tumor formation, blood clots, permanent blindness from improper eye injections, and spinal injuries. These clinics often charge tens of thousands of dollars for procedures with no scientific support, performed by individuals without appropriate training. My advice: avoid these unregulated stem cell clinics. If a stem cell treatment interests you, ask your doctor whether there is a legitimate clinical trial that you could join.

Metformin and Longevity

Metformin is a decades-old, inexpensive, and generally safe diabetes medication with an intriguing side finding: diabetic patients taking it appear to develop fewer age-related diseases than expected—including cancer and cardiovascular disease. Complicating conclusions about this correlation is the fact that people who take metformin differ from those who do not in many ways, and correlation does not establish causation. Animal studies show anti-aging effects in some models and no effect in others. The FDA does not recognize aging as a disease, which complicates the path to approval for any drug intended to slow it.

The TAME Trial

The TAME trial (Targeting Aging with Metformin) is a large, properly designed randomized controlled trial (RCT) testing whether metformin delays age-related diseases in non-diabetic older adults. It is one of the most important longevity trials underway. The drug causes common side effects—nausea, diarrhea. Until TAME results are available, the evidence for using metformin in non-diabetics to slow aging is not sufficient to recommend it.

Omega-3s, Vitamin D, and Exercise

Omega-3 fatty acids—found in fatty fish, walnuts, and flaxseed, and in the Mediterranean diet—have genuine cardiovascular and anti-inflammatory benefits when obtained through food. They may also slow telomere shortening and support brain-derived neurotrophic factor (BDNF), which promotes the growth and survival of brain cells (see Chapter 6). A well-designed clinical trial (DO-HEALTH, published in the British Medical Journal) found that the combination of 1 gram of omega-3s daily, 2,000 IU of vitamin D3, and 30 minutes of strength training three times per week reduced cancer risk, lowered the risk of frailty and falls, and decreased heart attack risk. This combination is notable because it is safe, inexpensive, and the exercise component alone may deliver significant benefit.

NAD+ Supplements and Cellular Energy

Every cell in your body runs on ATP—adenosine triphosphate, the molecule that stores and delivers energy for virtually every biological process. Think of it as a rechargeable battery: it gets "spent" after powering muscle contractions, heartbeats, and nerve signals, and the mitochondria—the cell's energy factories—continuously recharge it using oxygen, glucose, and fats. As we age, mitochondria become less efficient at this process. NAD+ (nicotinamide adenine dinucleotide) is a molecule essential to mitochondrial energy production, and its levels decline significantly with age. This decline has made NAD+ a popular target for anti-aging supplements.

Efficacy of NAD+ Supplements

The most common NAD+ supplements—NR (nicotinamide riboside) and NMN (nicotinamide mononucleotide)—are marketed with the assumption that they are converted into NAD+. They do appear to raise blood NAD+ levels in humans, which sounds promising. The problem is that higher blood NAD+ levels have not been reliably shown to translate into meaningful clinical benefits. Human trials are short, small, and have produced inconsistent results; a few small studies show modest improvements in grip strength and walking speed, but nothing definitive. A meaningful theoretical concern: cancer cells are metabolically very active and depend heavily on NAD+ for their rapid growth. Supplementing NAD+ precursors could hypothetically accelerate the growth of undetected tumors. Given the high cost, weak evidence, and this theoretical risk, I would not recommend these supplements. If you choose to use them, discuss it with your doctor first.

Lifestyle Versus NAD+ Supplements

Exercise—particularly strength training—is the most reliable and proven way to support mitochondrial function and NAD+

metabolism. A nutrient-rich diet, adequate sleep, and maintaining a healthy weight all contribute as well. These approaches carry no cancer risk, cost nothing beyond time, and deliver a wide range of additional benefits that no supplement can match.

Ketogenic Diets and Ketone Supplements

The ketogenic diet—very high fat, very low carbohydrate—forces the body to burn fat for fuel rather than glucose, producing molecules called ketones. This diet may produce meaningful short-term weight loss, but its long-term health profile compares poorly to a Mediterranean diet. Side effects include flu-like symptoms during the initial transition, fatty liver disease, elevated LDL cholesterol, significant fiber deficiency (which increases risks for constipation, colon cancer, and diverticulitis), and possibly increased cancer risk from chronic inflammation. In long-term mouse studies, ketogenic diets have been associated with shorter, not longer, lifespan. Ketone supplements have a specific legitimate use: managing drug-resistant epilepsy in children. Claims that ketone supplements extend longevity or improve health in adults remain unproven. Separately, very low-protein ketogenic diets are sometimes promoted for kidney disease; based on my review of the evidence, this approach is unlikely to slow kidney function decline and carries serious nutritional risks.

Peptide Therapy

Peptides are short chains of amino acids—smaller versions of proteins—that can act as signaling molecules in the body.

Peptide therapy includes the well-studied and FDA-approved GLP-1 receptor agonists—semaglutide (Ozempic, Wegovy), tirzepatide (Mounjaro, Zepbound)—which have strong evidence for weight loss and metabolic benefit. These peptides are not the concern. The concern is unregulated "research chemical" peptides sold online, often labeled "Not for Human Consumption" to circumvent FDA oversight. BPC-157, TB-500, Semax, and combined growth hormone-releasing peptides (CJC/Ipamorelin) fall into this category. Products labeled "not for human consumption" can contain heavy metals, bacterial contamination, and inaccurate dosages. Peptides that stimulate cell growth and new blood vessel formation—like BPC-157—may also accelerate the growth of undetected tumors. Growth hormone boosters can cause fluid retention, hand and foot swelling, and carpal tunnel-like nerve compression. I recommend avoiding all unregulated research chemical peptides. If you are curious about a specific peptide, ask your doctor whether a legitimate clinical trial exists for it.

Senolytics

As cells age and their telomeres shorten, many enter senescence—meaning they stop dividing but do not die. They become what researchers colorfully call "zombie cells": lingering in tissues, leaking inflammatory signals that damage neighboring healthy cells. The body's normal cellular cleanup system (autophagy) slows with age, allowing these zombie cells to accumulate. Senolytics are drugs designed to selectively eliminate these zombie cells, with the goal of reducing the inflammation they cause. The concept is compelling and the mouse evidence is strong—clearing senescent cells in aged mice extends lifespan and improves physical function. Human data is early and mixed. A combination of dasatinib (a leukemia drug) and quercetin (a chemical produced by some plants)—known as D+Q—has shown reductions in inflammatory markers and senescent cell counts in small human studies. D+Q is under investigation in clinical trials for diabetic kidney disease and pulmonary fibrosis. The dasatinib part of D+Q carries significant risks as a powerful chemotherapy drug. This combination should only be considered under strict medical supervision in a research setting.

Dangers of Senolytics

The risks of using senolytics outside of clinical trials are significant and underappreciated. Cellular senescence is not only a sign of aging—it is also one of the body's defenses against cancer. Senescent cells cannot divide, which means they cannot become tumors. Eliminating them indiscriminately removes that protection. In younger people especially, use of senolytics could theoretically increase cancer risk. The commercial senolytic products available online—sold in multi-day pulsed protocols (2 days per month, weekly, or daily)—are not regulated by the FDA for safety or efficacy. There is no guarantee of purity, potency, or accurate dosing. Experts in the field are essentially unanimous: do not use senolytics outside of a clinical trial. The science is promising; the products available today are not ready.

Should You Consider Fasting to Prolong Your Life?

Caloric restriction—reducing intake by roughly a third—extends lifespan by up to 30 percent in mice and rats, making it one of the most reproducible longevity findings in animal research. The human picture is less clear. Genetics appear to matter enormously: in some mouse strains, caloric restriction shortens rather than lengthens life. And severe restriction in older adults risks muscle loss, nutrient deficiency, and impaired immune function—consequences that could reduce rather than extend healthy years. Intermittent fasting—time-restricted eating rather than prolonged total fasts—may have benefits. Some studies show improvements in insulin sensitivity, blood sugar, and cholesterol, along with modest weight loss. But no long-term randomized trial has shown that intermittent fasting extends human lifespan. My recommendation: I do not suggest fasting purely for longevity. If supervised weight-loss fasting is part of a plan developed with your doctor, that is a different conversation.

Ozone Therapy

Ozone (O_3)—the molecule that forms the atmospheric layer protecting Earth from ultraviolet radiation—is also the primary component of smog and a known lung irritant. The FDA classifies ozone as a toxic gas with no proven medical applications. Proponents of ozone therapy claim it stimulates oxygen use, boosts immunity, and kills pathogens. The evidence does not support these claims, and the risks are real: even small amounts of inhaled ozone damage lung tissue. Ozone injections carry the additional risk of gas embolism—a bubble of gas that enters the bloodstream and can block vessels—potentially causing stroke, heart attack, or death. This is one of the clearest cases where serious risks are documented without any proven benefits. Avoid all forms of ozone therapy.

Plasma Exchange Therapy

Therapeutic plasma exchange—removing the liquid portion of the blood (plasma) and returning replacement fluids and the patient's blood cells—is a legitimate medical procedure used for certain diseases like myasthenia gravis and Guillain-Barré syndrome. Its use as an anti-aging treatment is a different matter entirely, with no solid scientific support. The theoretical idea is to remove pro-aging proteins circulating in older blood. The procedure carries real risks: low blood pressure, low calcium, and infection or bleeding at the catheter site. There is also preliminary evidence suggesting it may accelerate rather than slow aging. Undergoing a medical procedure with these risks for a benefit that has not been demonstrated is not a reasonable trade-off. Avoid plasma exchange for anti-aging purposes.

Will a Dose of Young Blood Help You Age More Slowly?

Animal research has shown that circulating young blood through older mice improves mental function and extends lifespan, generating interest in whether something similar might work in humans. The honest answer is: we do not know yet. The scientific question being pursued is whether specific proteins in young blood—or the absence of certain proteins in old blood—

are responsible for the effect, and whether those factors can be isolated and used safely. That research is ongoing and legitimate. Clinics offering young blood transfusions now—for significant fees, to healthy adults—are ahead of the evidence. The risks of transfusion (infection, immune reactions, transfusion-related complications) are real and well-documented. The benefits are not established in humans. Avoid unregulated transfusion clinics.

Hyperbaric Oxygen Therapy (HBOT)

Hyperbaric oxygen therapy—breathing pure oxygen in a pressurized chamber—has legitimate, well-established medical uses: treating decompression sickness in divers, non-healing diabetic foot wounds, carbon monoxide poisoning, and certain infections. Insurance covers it for these indications. Its use as an anti-aging or longevity treatment is based on a handful of small studies without control groups—a fundamental methodological flaw that makes the results uninterpretable. Side effects include claustrophobia and anxiety, and at higher pressures, ear and lung damage. I recommend HBOT only for its proven medical indications. For everything else, the cost, inconvenience, and risk are not justified by the evidence.

Red Light Therapy

Red light therapy uses specific wavelengths of low-energy light directed at the skin. The theoretical mechanism is that the light is absorbed by an enzyme in mitochondria (the cell's energy factories), potentially boosting their energy output. Small, short-term studies—with highly variable light parameters—suggest it may modestly improve skin appearance (reducing fine lines, improving texture), reduce localized joint pain, and possibly stimulate hair growth. No human trial has shown it extends lifespan. The risks are generally low but real: staring directly into the light can damage the eyes, and in people taking photosensitizing medications such as retinoids (see Chapter 11), it can cause chemical burns. For those with active cancer, there is a theoretical concern that stimulating mitochondrial activity could accelerate tumor growth. Red light therapy is not dangerous enough to warrant a strong warning, but it is not proven enough to recommend without reservation. If you think it might help with pain or skin appearance, the risk is low—but protect your eyes and discuss it with your doctor first.

Cold Plunges and Sauna

Sauna research comes primarily from Finland, where regular sauna use is deeply embedded in the culture. Long-term studies of large populations of Finns have produced consistently positive findings: frequent sauna use (four to seven times per week) is associated with lower rates of fatal cardiovascular disease, reduced blood pressure, lower risk of Alzheimer's dementia, and decreased muscle and joint pain. These are associations rather than controlled trials, so causality cannot be established—sauna users may differ from non-users in important ways. Still, the consistency of the findings is worth taking seriously, particularly for cardiovascular health. Cold plunge research is much thinner. The practice of alternating intense heat with cold immersion places significant stress on the cardiovascular system. Combined with alcohol—common in some contexts—or in people with cardiovascular disease, it can be dangerous. Discuss with your doctor before starting either practice, especially if you have any heart or blood pressure concerns.

Should You Monitor Your Glucose Levels and Heart Rate Variability?

Continuous glucose monitors (CGMs) have well-established benefit for people with diabetes: they reduce dangerous blood sugar swings and improve management. For healthy individuals without diabetes, the picture is different. Normal blood sugar fluctuates after meals in ways that are entirely expected and require no intervention; watching those fluctuations in real time has the potential to create anxiety and an unhealthy preoccupation with food. Heart rate variability (HRV)—the variation in time between heartbeats—is a marker of autonomic (sympathetic/parasympathetic) nervous system health that declines with age. Higher HRV correlates with fitness and has some predictive value for cardiac risk after a heart attack. It can be a useful training guide for athletes. For most people, however, the evidence that monitoring HRV and adjusting behavior based on it improves outcomes is thin. The broader risk of intensive self-monitoring is that constant data can produce anxiety and decision fatigue rather than useful insight. The lifestyle fundamentals discussed throughout this book are a better investment of your attention than wearable monitoring devices.

Does Altering the Gut Microbiome Affect Longevity?

The gut microbiome's influence on aging is one of the most scientifically credible frontiers in longevity research. The most striking evidence comes from microbiome transplant experiments: transferring the gut microbiome from young fish or mice into older ones extends lifespan and improves physical function. The reverse experiment—transplanting an aged microbiome into young animals—causes intestinal leakage and elevated systemic inflammation, the hallmarks of inflammaging (see Chapter 16). Some people who live beyond 100 have distinctively diverse and resilient microbiomes, though whether that is a cause or a consequence of their longevity is not yet known. This is one area where actionable guidance exists right now: a varied plant-rich diet, fermented foods, and avoiding unnecessary antibiotics and PPIs all support microbiome health (see Chapters 2 and 14). The specific tools to "program" the microbiome for longevity remain under development, but the dietary foundations are well-established.

Total Body CT and Whole-Body MRI — "Longevity Scans"

The idea behind total-body imaging for healthy adults is appealing: catch problems before they cause symptoms, when treatment is most likely to succeed. CT scans are highly sensitive at detecting early tumors in the lungs, kidneys, and liver; they can identify coronary artery calcification (CAC) and aortic aneurysms (see Chapters 3 and 4); and knowing your calcium score may help guide decisions about cholesterol-lowering medication and lifestyle changes. Early detection of a malignancy significantly improves surgical outcomes.

The case for screening has some potential benefit, but the medical community generally cautions against total-body CT for healthy, asymptomatic individuals, for well-documented reasons. A single total-body CT delivers ionizing radiation equivalent to roughly 100 to 150 chest X-rays. Repeated scans over years or decades statistically increase the risk of radiation-induced cancers, which somewhat undermines the longevity purpose. The more universal problem is incidentalomas (see Chapter 20). CT scans are so sensitive that they routinely find small nodules, cysts, or shadows that are almost certainly benign but cannot be definitively proven so without further investigation. A "spot on your lung" finding triggers follow-up CT scans, PET scans, and sometimes biopsies or surgery—for what often turns out to be a harmless scar from a childhood infection. The anxiety this generates is real and can persist for months. CT also has blind spots: it can miss certain pancreatic, stomach, and ovarian cancers and small lesions, which can create a false sense of security.

Whole-body MRI (WBMRI) is an increasingly popular alternative, promoted primarily because it uses no ionizing radiation and can therefore be repeated annually. MRI's superior soft-tissue contrast makes it excellent for detecting solid tumors in the pancreas, prostate, kidneys, and liver at very early stages, and it can identify silent strokes, early neurodegenerative changes, and brain aneurysms before symptoms appear. The absence of radiation is a genuine advantage. The drawbacks are significant. WBMRI produces even more incidentalomas than

CT—more "bright spots" and "shadows" requiring expensive, stressful, and sometimes invasive follow-up. Cost is a major barrier: most longevity-focused WBMRI clinics operate outside insurance coverage, charging $2,500 to $5,000 per scan. MRI is not as good as low-dose CT for detecting early lung nodules—the leading cause of cancer death in smokers and ex-smokers. A standard WBMRI does not generate a coronary calcium score, and it cannot replace colonoscopy for detecting precancerous colon polyps.

The bottom line for most healthy adults is to use targeted screening tests with established evidence—low-dose lung CT for current or former heavy smokers, coronary calcium scoring for cardiovascular risk, colonoscopy for colon cancer prevention. These approaches are better supported than a total-body scan that finds everything, including things that were better left unfound. If you are considering a "longevity scan," discuss your specific risk profile (strong family history of pancreatic or other cancers) with your doctor before committing to it.

Experimental Therapies and Frailty

Many of the interventions in this chapter target frailty—the syndrome of declining strength, slow walking speed, low physical activity, unintentional weight loss, and exhaustion that predicts poor health outcomes in older adults. Frailty is not a normal or inevitable part of aging. It is a medical syndrome that can be prevented and, in many cases, reversed. The most effective treatments are not experimental: adequate protein intake, strength training, and staying mentally and socially active have stronger evidence for preventing and reversing frailty than any supplement or clinic procedure discussed in this chapter. Before spending money on any experimental therapy, apply two tests: has it been studied in a properly designed RCT in humans, and has that trial been independently replicated?

Conclusion

The $75 billion longevity market has an enormous incentive to sell hope to people who are beginning to notice their own aging and feel the urgency of doing something about it. That is a completely human response—and the industry is expertly designed to meet it. The most important skill this chapter can offer is a framework for evaluating claims before spending money or accepting risk: Is there an RCT in humans? Who funded it? Has it been independently replicated? What are the known risks? Is the product or procedure regulated? After applying this framework honestly, only a handful of interventions emerge as worth recommending: the omega-3/vitamin D/exercise combination, regular sauna use, and a microbiome-supporting diet. Most of the rest warrant waiting for better evidence. Many should be avoided outright. And the lifestyle foundations covered throughout this book—exercise, diet, sleep, and social connection—remain the highest-evidence, lowest-risk longevity interventions available, at any price.

Chapter 20:

Artificial Intelligence (AI) and the Future of Medicine

ARTIFICIAL INTELLIGENCE IS ALREADY reshaping medicine in ways that matter for anyone reading this book—and the pace of change is accelerating. This chapter covers what AI is currently doing for aging patients, where it is headed in the near term, and what the longer-range possibilities look like. The core promise is a shift from reactive medicine—treating disease after it has already caused damage—to predictive and preventive medicine that keeps people healthy longer. The chapter also covers AI's real limitations and risks, which deserve honest attention alongside the genuine excitement.

Current AI Applications for Health Span and Lifespan

The traditional trajectory of aging involves a long, gradual decline in health over years or decades before death. One of AI's most compelling potential contributions is compressing that decline: keeping health on a high plateau for as long as possible, with a much shorter period of serious decline at the end of life. Several current applications point in this direction. AI can estimate your biological age—how fast your body is aging relative to your calendar age—by analyzing DNA methylation patterns in blood (epigenetic clocks, see Chapter 8) and, more recently, facial features. AI also helps doctors navigate complex cases by combining information from patient records with up-to-date medical literature to suggest diagnoses and personalized treatment options. It is being used to predict the onset of diseases like Alzheimer's and type 2 diabetes years before symptoms appear, potentially opening a window for prevention. AI image analysis of X-rays, MRIs, and CT scans has reached or exceeded the accuracy of specialist radiologists in several domains, and cancer detection algorithms can identify suspicious findings in mammograms, lung scans, and skin images two to three years before they would typically become symptomatic. One important caution applies to imaging AI: the same sensitivity that finds early tumors also finds incidentalomas—benign findings that look suspicious—leading to follow-up procedures, patient anxiety, and in some cases unnecessary surgery (see Chapter 19).

AI and Digital Biomarkers

Wearable devices—smartwatches, continuous glucose monitors, blood pressure cuffs—already generate enormous amounts of physiological data. AI makes that data clinically useful by detecting patterns that would be invisible to any individual reviewing numbers manually. In hospital settings, AI monitoring has shown particular promise in identifying sepsis—life-threatening uncontrolled infection—hours before clinical signs appear. Earlier recognition translates directly into faster treatment and better survival. For individuals outside the hospital, AI-integrated wearables are increasingly capable of flagging atrial fibrillation (see Chapter 4), abnormal blood pressure patterns, and high or low glucose levels in real time, alerting both the wearer and their clinician before a crisis develops.

AI and Drug Development

Drug development has historically been a decade-long, enormously expensive process with a very high failure rate. AI is compressing the timeline. It can identify promising compounds in months rather than years and filter out likely failures before costly clinical trials begin. AI-identified drug candidates are already entering human trials for conditions ranging from rare diseases to cancer. In the longevity space specifically, AI is being used to screen for compounds that clear the senescent "zombie cells" (senolytics—discussed in Chapter 19). Beyond discovery, AI helps with medication adherence: by analyzing prescription refill patterns, medication histories, and socioeconomic factors, to identify patients at high risk of missing doses. It can trigger targeted outreach before a gap in treatment causes harm.

AI Chatbots and Clinical Documentation

AI-powered conversational tools—chatbots and virtual assistants—are expanding access to health information and support in meaningful ways. They can answer patient questions around the clock in plain language, provide mental health support in communities with few mental health providers, and conduct structured follow-ups after procedures or new prescriptions to catch side effects and adherence problems early. One of the highest-impact near-term applications is an AI that listens to a doctor-patient conversation and automatically generates the clinical note. This reduces the documentation burden that has become a leading driver of physician burnout, allowing doctors to give their full attention to the patient in front of them rather than to a computer screen. Several major health systems have begun deploying this technology, with strong early results for both clinician satisfaction and note quality.

AI in Surgery

AI-assisted robotic surgery has moved from novelty to mainstream practice in a number of specialties. Robotic systems provide surgeons with magnified, high-resolution three-dimensional views of the operative field and filter out hand tremor, enabling more precise movements than the human hand alone can achieve. In prostate cancer surgery, AI can superimpose the tumor location and the critical nerve bundles—which control continence and erectile function—directly onto the surgeon's view, helping preserve function while ensuring complete cancer removal. In joint replacement, AI analyzes the patient's specific anatomy from preoperative imaging to generate a customized surgical plan, improving implant fit and alignment. The evidence to date suggests AI-assisted surgery reduces certain complication rates and shortens recovery time. It does not eliminate the need for human skill and judgment—it augments them.

AI, Health Equity, and the Developing World

The transformative potential of AI in medicine may not be evenly distributed, and the gap could widen health disparities rather than close them. AI diagnostic systems perform only as well as the data they were trained on. Systems trained primarily on patients from high-income countries or specific ethnic populations can perform significantly worse for everyone else. Skin cancer detection algorithms trained on lighter skin tones have shown substantially lower accuracy in identifying melanomas on darker skin—a dangerous failure in exactly the populations with the least access to specialist dermatology. The World Economic Forum has estimated that AI-driven medicine could exclude up to five billion people in lower-income countries where training data, infrastructure, and regulatory frameworks lag far behind. Correcting this requires intentional diversity in the datasets used to train medical AI.

Disadvantages and Risks of AI in Medicine

The limitations and risks of AI in medicine deserve the same honest attention as its promise. The doctor-patient relationship depends on something more than accurate diagnosis—it depends on trust, empathy, and the sense of being heard. Over-reliance on AI can interfere with that therapeutic relationship. Another concern is that doctors who train with AI handling diagnosis and documentation from the start of their careers may not develop the clinical intuition that becomes essential when technology fails, is unavailable, or if the AI encounters a situation outside its training data. AI "hallucinations"—confidently stated errors—

are a documented problem in large language model systems, including medical ones. AI has fabricated medical references, invented drug interactions, and generated clinical summaries that sound authoritative but contain factual errors. Any AI system used for medical purposes requires human oversight and verification, not blind trust. Cybersecurity is a serious and underappreciated risk: researchers have demonstrated that AI diagnostic systems can be fooled by subtle alterations to medical images, potentially causing misdiagnoses. Healthcare infrastructure, already a major target for hackers, becomes more vulnerable as it becomes more AI-dependent.

The Future: Artificial General Intelligence (AGI)

The AI systems in use today were trained for specific tasks. Artificial General Intelligence (AGI) refers to a hypothetical system with flexible, human-like reasoning that can learn from experience, draw causal conclusions, and apply knowledge it was not specifically trained on. No AGI system exists yet, and researchers disagree about when or whether it will. If AGI is achieved, its medical implications would be profound. A system that could simultaneously analyze a patient's genome, microbiome, real-time physiological data, full medical history, and the entire published medical literature—and update its reasoning as new evidence emerged—could potentially detect disease risks, generate diagnostic hypotheses, and recommend treatment plans that no individual clinician could match. It could also be used to produce harmful pathogens and to create havoc for the medical establishment. The questions AGI raises—about accountability, trust, the role of human judgment, and what it means to be cared for by another person—are as important as the technical capabilities themselves.

Artificial Superintelligence (ASI)

Beyond AGI, theorists describe Artificial Superintelligence (ASI): a system that would exceed the combined cognitive capacity of all humans and could improve its own capabilities faster than humans could comprehend or control. ASI remains firmly in the realm of speculation—there is no scientific consensus on whether it is achievable, on what timescale, or what it would mean in practice. The potential benefits imagined for ASI are extraordinary: solving aging, eradicating disease, unlocking clean fusion energy. The risks—of a system whose goals and values may not align with human well-being—are taken seriously by many AI researchers.

Conclusion

AI can advance the practice of medicine through earlier disease detection, better-matched treatments, more accessible health information, and reduced barriers in underserved communities. The risks—hallucinations, bias against underrepresented populations, erosion of the human dimensions of care, and cybersecurity vulnerabilities—are equally real and require ongoing attention from clinicians, regulators, and patients alike. The most important thing to understand about AI in medicine is that it is a tool. The best outcomes will come from AI and clinicians working together. That partnership—not AI replacing doctors—will be the future of medicine.

Acknowledgments

THROUGHOUT MY LIFE AS a physician, I have found deep satisfaction in helping patients, friends, and family navigate their medical challenges. I never expected to reach people around the world with answers to medical questions and up-to-date guidance on health topics. James Fabin provided that opportunity through my appearances on his YouTube channel, DadviceTV. James also gave my first book a platform it might never otherwise have found. His generosity and his genuine commitment to providing evidence-based science to his audience have served as both a role model and a motivator for me. I owe a particular debt to the colleagues, mentors, and collaborators who have helped shape my thinking on dialysis timing and the broader practice of nephrology and internal medicine. I am especially grateful to those colleagues who supported me when I challenged conventional thinking when the evidence supported me doing so. I want to thank my son David for his helpful ideas and edits and my partner, Alice , or her steady support.

Diana Wade of Diana Wade Designs created the cover and interior layout for this book, as well as for my first book. Her design sensibility and her patience with revisions made the finished books far better than they would have been otherwise.

I am grateful to my children and grandchildren, who are a constant source of perspective on what matters in a life well lived.

Watching them grow has reminded me, more than any clinical experience, that health span is ultimately measured in the time we have to spend with the people we love.

Key References

The references below are listed by chapter as suggested further reading. They are not linked to specific statements in the text; rather, they represent the landmark studies, clinical guidelines, and authoritative reviews that inform the topics discussed in each chapter.

Chapter 1 — Exercise as the Modern "Fountain of Youth"

1. Bull FC, Al-Ansari SS, Biddle S, et al. World Health Organization 2020 guidelines on physical activity and sedentary behavior. Br J Sports Med. 2020;54(24):1451-1462. — International consensus on activity doses for adults of all ages.

2. Lee IM, Shiroma EJ, Lobelo F, et al. Effect of physical inactivity on major non- communicable diseases worldwide: an analysis of burden of disease and life expectancy. Lancet. 2012;380(9838):219-229. — Landmark paper quantifying life-expectancy cost of inactivity; supports the "7 minutes of life per minute of exercise" framing.

3. Paluch AE, Bajpai S, Bassett DR, et al. Daily steps and all-cause mortality: a meta-analysis of 15 international cohorts. Lancet Public Health. 2022;7(3):e219-e228. — Best contemporary evidence on step-count targets; supports the 7,000–9,000-step mortality benefit.

4. Garber CE, Blissmer B, Deschenes MR, et al; American

College of Sports Medicine. Quantity and quality of exercise for developing and maintaining cardiorespiratory, musculoskeletal, and neuromotor fitness in apparently healthy adults. Med Sci Sports Exerc. 2011;43(7):1334-1359. — ACSM position stand on exercise prescription; supports heart-rate-target and resistance-training sections.

5. Stamatakis E, Ahmadi MN, Friedenreich CM, et al. Vigorous intermittent lifestyle physical activity and mortality. Nat Med. 2022;28(12):2521-2529. — Supports the "exercise bursts versus any movement" section.

Chapter 2 — Your Weight, Diet, and Weight Loss Medications

1. Estruch R, Ros E, Salas-Salvadó J, et al. Primary prevention of cardiovascular disease with a Mediterranean diet supplemented with extra-virgin olive oil or nuts. N Engl J Med. 2018;378(25):e34. — The landmark RCT of the Mediterranean diet; central to the Mediterranean-diet section.

2. Wilding JPH, Batterham RL, Calanna S,et al; STEP 1 Study Group. Once-weeklysemaglutide in adults with overweight or obesity. N Engl J Med. 2021;384(11):989-1002. — Pivotal RCT for GLP-1 efficacy discussion.

3. Jastreboff AM, Aronne LJ, Ahmad NN, etal; SURMOUNT-1 Investigators. Tirzepatide once weekly for the treatment of obesity. N Engl J Med.2022;387(3):205-216. — Second major GLP-1 weight-loss trial.

4. Lincoff AM, Brown-Frandsen K, ColhounHM, et al; SELECT Trial Investigators. Semaglutide and cardiovascular outcomes in obesity without diabetes. NEngl J Med.

2023;389(24):2221-2232. —Supports the cardiovascular-benefit-of-weight-loss.

5. Monteiro CA, Cannon G, Levy RB, et al.Ultra-processed foods: what they are and how to identify them. Public Health Nutr.2019;22(5):936-941. — Foundation for the ultra-processed-foods section.

6. Hall KD, Ayuketah A, Brychta R, et al.Ultra-processed diets cause excess calorie intake and weight gain: an inpatient randomized controlled trial of ad libitum food intake. Cell Metab.2019;30(1):67-77.e3. — The NIH metabolic-ward study showing UPFs drive higher caloric intake; supports UPF harms.

7. Look AHEAD Research Group.Cardiovascular effects of intensive lifestyle intervention in type 2 diabetes. NEngl J Med. 2013;369(2):145-154. —Informs discussion of weight-loss and longevity.

Chapter 3 — Slowing Atherosclerosis: A Key to Lifespan and Health Span

1. SPRINT Research Group; Wright JT Jr, Williamson JD, Whelton PK, et al. A randomized trial of intensive versus standard blood-pressure control. N Engl J Med. 2015;373(22):2103-2116. — The SPRINT trial — foundational for the "target-120 mmHg systolic" recommendation.

2. Whelton PK, Carey RM, Aronow WS, et al. 2017 Guideline for the Prevention, Detection, Evaluation, and Management of High Blood Pressure in Adults. J Am Coll Cardiol. 2018;71(19):e127-e248. — Supports BP classification, measurement technique, and drug selection.

3. Grundy SM, Stone NJ, Bailey AL, et al. 2018 Guideline on the Management of Blood Cholesterol. J Am Coll Cardiol. 2019;73(24):e285-e350. — Basis for LDL- targeting recommendations and statin discussion.

4. Sabatine MS, Giugliano RP, Keech AC, et al; FOURIER Steering Committee and Investigators. Evolocumab and clinical outcomes in patients with cardiovascular disease. N Engl J Med. 2017;376(18):1713-1722. supports aggressive LDL-lowering discussion.

5. McNeil JJ, Wolfe R, Woods RL, et al; ASPREE Investigator Group. Effect of aspirin on cardiovascular events and bleeding in the healthy elderly. N Engl J Med. 2018;379(16):1509-1518. — Evidence against routine aspirin for primary prevention in older adults.

6. US Preventive Services Task Force; Davidson KW, Barry MJ, Mangione CM, et al. Aspirin use to prevent cardiovascular disease: US Preventive Services Task Force recommendation statement. JAMA. 2022;327(16):1577- 1584. — Current USPSTF aspirin recommendation.

7. GBD 2019 Risk Factors Collaborators. Global burden of 87 risk factors in 204 countries and territories, 1990–2019. Lancet. 2020;396(10258):1223-1249. — Global burden data on smoking and CVD risk factors.

Chapter 4 — Age-Related Heart Diseases

1. Joglar JA, Chung MK, Armbruster AL, et al. 2023 guideline for the diagnosis and management of atrial fibrillation. J Am Coll Cardiol. 2024;83(1):109-279. — Guideline for AF

diagnosis, rate/rhythm control, and anticoagulation.

2. Heidenreich PA, Bozkurt B, Aguilar D, et al. 2022 guideline for the management of heart failure. J Am Coll Cardiol. 2022;79(17):e263-e421. — Basis for HFpEF/HFrEF distinctions.

3. McMurray JJV, Solomon SD, Inzucchi SE, et al; DAPA-HF Trial Committees and Investigators. Dapagliflozin in patients with heart failure and reduced ejection fraction. N Engl J Med. 2019;381(21):1995-2008. — Supports SGLT2-in-HF discussion.

4. Kosiborod MN, Abildstrøm SZ, Borlaug BA, et al; STEP-HFpEF Trial Committees and Investigators. Semaglutide in patients with heart failure with preserved ejection fraction and obesity. N Engl J Med. 2023;389(12):1069-1084. — Supports the weight-loss-in-HF sections.

5. Marrouche NF, Brachmann J, Andresen D, et al; CASTLE-AF Investigators. Catheter ablation for atrial fibrillation with heart failure. N Engl J Med. 2018;378(5):417-427. — Ablation benefits in AF with HF.

6. Virani SS, Newby LK, Arnold SV, et al. 2023 Guideline for the Management of Patients With Chronic Coronary Disease. J Am Coll Cardiol. 2023;82(9):833-955. — Current chronic CAD guideline; angina management and secondary prevention.

Chapter 5 — Blood Vessel Disease of the Brain

1. Powers WJ, Rabinstein AA, Ackerson T, et al. Guidelines for the early management of patients with acute ischemic stroke. Stroke. 2019;50(12):e344-e418. — Acute-stroke guideline; supports tPA windows,

2. Kleindorfer DO, Towfighi A, Chaturvedi S, et al. 2021

Guideline for the Prevention of Stroke in Patients With Stroke and Transient Ischemic Attack. Stroke. 2021;52(7):e364-e467. — Secondary stroke prevention guideline.

3. Nogueira RG, Jadhav AP, Haussen DC, et al; DAWN Trial Investigators. Thrombectomy 6 to 24 hours after stroke with a mismatch between deficit and infarct. N Engl J Med. 2018;378(1):11-21. — Extended-window thrombectomy.

4. Meschia JF, Bushnell C, Boden-Albala B, et al. Guidelines for the primary prevention of stroke. Stroke. 2014;45(12):3754-3832. — Supports BP, lipids, and AF management for stroke prevention.

5. Hemphill JC 3rd, Greenberg SM, Anderson CS, et al. Guidelines for the management of spontaneous intracerebral hemorrhage. Stroke. 2015;46(7):2032-2060. — Intracerebral hemorrhage management guideline.

Chapter 6 — Maintaining Brain and Nervous System Function

1. Livingston G, Huntley J, Liu KY, et al. Dementia prevention, intervention, and care: 2024 report of the Lancet standing Commission. Lancet. 2024;404(10452):572-628. — ~45% of dementia potentially preventable. Essential citation.

2. Ngandu T, Lehtisalo J, Solomon A, et al. A 2 year multidomain intervention of diet, exercise, cognitive training, and vascular risk monitoring versus control to prevent cognitive decline in at-risk elderly people (FINGER). Lancet. 2015;385(9984):2255- 2263. — foundational lifestyle- intervention RCT for cognitive decline.

3. Lin FR, Pike JR, Albert MS, et al; ACHIEVE Collaborative Research Group. Hearing intervention versus health education

control to reduce cognitive decline in older adults with hearing loss in the USA (ACHIEVE): a multicenter, randomized controlled trial. Lancet. 2023;402(10404):786-797. — Hearing aids reduced cognitive decline 48% in at- risk older adults; supports hearing-loss- and-dementia discussion.

4. van Dyck CH, Swanson CJ, Aisen P, et al. Lecanemab in early Alzheimer's disease. N Engl J Med. 2023;388(1):9-21. — CLARITY-AD — pivotal lecanemab trial.

5. Pase MP, Himali JJ, Jacques PF, et al. Sugary beverage intake and preclinical Alzheimer's disease in the community. Alzheimers Dement. 2017;13(9):955-964. — Supports the dietary-risk discussion for cognitive health.

6. Holt-Lunstad J, Smith TB, Baker M, et al. Loneliness and social isolation as risk factors for mortality: a meta-analytic review. Perspect Psychol Sci. 2015;10(2):227-237. — Foundational meta-analysis on social connection and health; supports the social-engagement- and-cognition discussion (also Chapter 18).

Chapter 7 — How to Reverse Diabetes and Reduce Its Harmful Effects

1. American Diabetes Association Professional Practice Committee. Standards of Care in Diabetes—2025. Diabetes Care. 2025;48(Suppl 1):S1- S352. — Current ADA Standards of Care; the primary professional reference for all diabetes management questions.

2. Lean MEJ, Leslie WS, Barnes AC, et al. Primary care-led weight management for remission of type 2 diabetes (DiRECT): an open-label, cluster-randomized trial. Lancet.

2018;391(10120):541-551. — Landmark trial demonstrating diabetes remission through structured weight loss.

3. Zinman B, Wanner C, Lachin JM, et al; EMPA-REG OUTCOME Investigators. Empagliflozin, cardiovascular outcomes, and mortality in type 2 diabetes. N Engl J Med. 2015;373(22):2117-2128. — First SGLT2 cardiovascular outcomes trial.

4. Marso SP, Daniels GH, Brown-Frandsen K, et al; LEADER Steering Committee. Liraglutide and cardiovascular outcomes in type 2 diabetes. N Engl J Med. 2016;375(4):311-322. — Foundational GLP-1 CV outcomes trial in diabetes.

5. UK Prospective Diabetes Study (UKPDS) Group. Intensive blood-glucose control with sulphonylureas or insulin compared with conventional treatment and risk of complications in patients with type 2 diabetes (UKPDS 33). Lancet. 1998;352(9131):837-853. — UKPDS — the foundational diabetes outcomes trial; still widely cited for long-term complication

6. Mingrone G, Panunzi S, De Gaetano A, et al. Metabolic surgery versus conventional medical therapy in patients with type 2 diabetes: 10-year follow-up of an open-label, single-center, randomized controlled trial. Lancet. 2021;397(10271):293-304. — Long-term bariatric-surgery evidence for diabetes reversal.

7. Perkovic V, Jardine MJ, Neal B, et al; CREDENCE Trial Investigators. Canagliflozin and renal outcomes in type 2 diabetes and nephropathy. N Engl J Med. 2019;380(24):2295-2306. — SGLT2 inhibitor renal protection in diabetes; supports complication-prevention discussion.

Chapter 8 — Genes Are Not Destiny

1. International Human Genome Sequencing Consortium. Finishing the euchromatic sequence of the human genome. Nature. 2004;431(7011):931- 945. — Completion of the Human Genome Project; foundational for genetics chapter.

2. Jinek M, Chylinski K, Fonfara I, Hauer M, Doudna JA, Charpentier E. A programmable dual-RNA-guided DNA endonuclease in adaptive bacterial immunity. Science. 2012;337(6096):816- 821. — Foundational CRISPR-Cas9 paper (Doudna/Charpentier, Nobel Prize 2020).

3. Frangoul H, Altshuler D, Cappellini MD, et al. CRISPR-Cas9 gene editing for sickle cell disease and β-thalassemia. N Engl J Med. 2021;384(3):252-260. — First-in-human CRISPR therapeutic success (exa-cel/Casgevy, FDA-approved 2023); supports CRISPR clinical- application section.

4. Jumper J, Evans R, Pritzel A, et al. Highly accurate protein structure prediction with AlphaFold. Nature. 2021;596(7873):583-589. — AlphaFold — Nobel-Prize-winning work on protein folding; supports protein-folding and AI-in-genetics sections.

5. Khera AV, Chaffin M, Aragam KG, et al. Genome-wide polygenic scores for common diseases identify individuals with risk equivalent to monogenic mutations. Nat Genet. 2018;50(9):1219-1224. — Landmark polygenic risk score paper; supports the genetic-screening discussion.

6. Horvath S, Raj K. DNA methylation- based biomarkers and the epigenetic clock theory of ageing. Nat Rev Genet. 2018;19(6):371-384. — Foundational review on epigenetic

clocks; directly supports the epigenetics section.

Chapter 9 — Lifestyle Choices Can Reduce Your Risk of Cancer

1. World Cancer Research Fund/American Institute for Cancer Research. Diet, Nutrition, Physical Activity and Cancer: a Global Perspective. Continuous Update Project Expert Report 2018. — authoritative synthesis of lifestyle and cancer evidence; the single most comprehensive source for this chapter.

2. Rumgay H, Murphy N, Ferrari P, Soerjomataram I. Alcohol and cancer: epidemiology and biological mechanisms. Nutrients. 2021;13(9):3173. — Supports the alcohol-and-cancer discussion.

3. National Lung Screening Trial Research Team. Reduced lung-cancer mortality with low-dose computed tomographic screening. N Engl J Med. 2011;365(5):395-409. — Foundational lung-cancer screening trial; supports LDCT-screening discussion.

4. US Preventive Services Task Force; Davidson KW, Barry MJ, Mangione CM, et al. Screening for colorectal cancer: US Preventive Services Task Force recommendation statement. JAMA. 2021;325(19):1965-1977. — Current USPSTF colorectal cancer screening recommendation (screening now starts at 45).

5. Siegel RL, Giaquinto AN, Jemal A. Cancer statistics, 2024. CA Cancer J Clin. 2024;74(1):12-49. — Annual ACS cancer statistics.

6. International Agency for Research on Cancer. List of Classifications. IARC Monographs on the Identification of

Carcinogenic Hazards to Humans. Volumes 1-136. Lyon, France: IARC. — Authoritative carcinogen classifications for workplace/ environmental carcinogen discussion.

7. Rebbeck TR, Burns-White K, Chan AT, et al. Precision prevention and early detection of cancer: fundamental principles. Cancer Discov. 2018;8(7):803- 811. — Framework for cancer prevention by risk factor; supports lifestyle- modification discussion.

Chapter 10 — Your Muscles, Bones, and Joints

1. Cruz-Jentoft AJ, Bahat G, Bauer J, et al; Writing Group for the European Working Group on Sarcopenia in Older People 2 (EWGSOP2). Sarcopenia: revised European consensus on definition and diagnosis. Age Ageing. 2019;48(1):16-31. — Consensus sarcopenia definition; foundational for sarcopenia and muscle- loss discussion.

2. Bauer J, Biolo G, Cederholm T, et al. Evidence-based recommendations for optimal dietary protein intake in older people: a position paper from the PROT- AGE Study Group. J Am Med Dir Assoc. 2013;14(8):542-559. — Consensus on protein intake in older adults; supports protein recommendation (1.0–1.2 g/kg).

3. US Preventive Services Task Force; Curry SJ, Krist AH, Owens DK, et al. Screening for osteoporosis to prevent fractures: US Preventive Services Task Force recommendation statement. JAMA. 2018;319(24):2521-2531. — USPSTF osteoporosis screening guidance.

4. Fransen M, McConnell S, Harmer AR, Van der Esch M,

Simic M, Bennell KL. Exercise for osteoarthritis of the knee. Cochrane Database Syst Rev. 2015;(1):CD004376. — Cochrane review on exercise for knee OA; supports exercise-as-OA-treatment section.

5. Qaseem A, Wilt TJ, McLean RM, et al; Clinical Guidelines Committee of the American College of Physicians. Noninvasive treatments for acute, subacute, and chronic low back pain: A clinical practice guideline from the American College of Physicians. Ann Intern Med. 2017;166(7):514-530. — ACP low back pain guideline; supports low- back-pain section.

6. Sihvonen R, Paavola M, Malmivaara A, et al; Finnish Degenerative Meniscal Lesion Study (FIDELITY) Group. Arthroscopic partial meniscectomy versus sham surgery for a degenerative meniscal tear. N Engl J Med. 2013;369(26):2515-2524. — Landmark trial showing no benefit of arthroscopy for degenerative meniscus tears; supports "orthopedic procedures of questionable value" section.

Chapter 11 — Understanding Skin Care and Hair Health as We Age

1. Kligman LH, Kligman AM. The nature of photoaging: its prevention and repair. Photodermatol. 1986;3(4):215-227. — Foundational photoaging paper; still cited for the basic mechanism.

2. Mukherjee S, Date A, Patravale V, Korting HC, Roeder A, Weindl G. Retinoids in the treatment of skin aging: an overview of clinical efficacy and safety. Clin Interv Aging. 2006;1(4):327-348. — Overview of retinoid evidence; supports retinoid section.

3. Bissett DL, Oblong JE, Berge CA. Niacinamide: A B vitamin that improves aging facial skin appearance. Dermatol Surg. 2005;31:860-865. — Foundational niacinamide skin-aging trial.

4. Pullar JM, Carr AC, Vissers MCM. The roles of vitamin C in skin health. Nutrients. 2017;9(8):866. — Supports vitamin C section.

5. Gupta AK, Foley KA, Mays RR, Shear NH, Piguet V. Monotherapy for treatment of androgenetic alopecia: network meta- analysis of finasteride, dutasteride, minoxidil, and tofacitinib. J Eur Acad Dermatol Venereol. 2022;36(4):571-584. — Meta-analysis supporting the hair-loss section.

6. Papakonstantinou E, Roth M, Karakiulakis G. Hyaluronic acid: a key molecule in skin aging. Dermatoendocrinol. 2012;4(3):253-258. — Foundational review on hyaluronic acid in skin.

Chapter 12 — Hormone Therapy and Aging

1. "The 2022 Hormone Therapy Position Statement of The North American Menopause Society" Advisory Panel. The 2022 Hormone Therapy Position Statement of The North American Menopause Society. Menopause. 2022;29(7):767-794. — Current NAMS menopause HT position — the authoritative source for HRT discussion.

2. Rossouw JE, Anderson GL, Prentice RL, et al; Writing Group for the Women's Health Initiative Investigators. Risks and benefits of estrogen plus progestin in healthy postmenopausal women. JAMA. 2002;288(3):321-333. — Original WHI HT

publication — essential historical/background reference.

3. Hodis HN, Mack WJ, Henderson VW, et al; ELITE Research Group. Vascular effects of early versus late postmenopausal treatment with estradiol. N Engl J Med. 2016;374(13):1221-1231. — Foundational for the "timing hypothesis" of HRT.

4. Snyder PJ, Bhasin S, Cunningham GR, et al; Testosterone Trials Investigators. Effects of testosterone treatment in older men. N Engl J Med. 2016;374(7):611-624. — T-Trials — foundational testosterone therapy RCTs in older men.

5. Lincoff AM, Bhasin S, Flevaris P, et al; TRAVERSE Study Investigators. Cardiovascular safety of testosterone- replacement therapy. N Engl J Med. 2023;389(2):107-117. — TRAVERSE — the definitive CV safety trial of TRT.

6. Ross DS, Burch HB, Cooper DS, et al. 2016 American Thyroid Association guidelines for diagnosis and management of hyperthyroidism and other causes of thyrotoxicosis. Thyroid. 2016;26(10):1343- 1421. — ATA thyroid guideline; supports the thyroid section.

7. Centers for Disease Control and Prevention. Sexually Transmitted Infections Treatment Guidelines, 2021. MMWR Recomm Rep. 2021;70(4):1-187. — Supports the "STI risk in older adults" section.

Chapter 13 — Your Eyes and Ears as You Age

1. Lin FR, Pike JR, Albert MS, et al. Hearing intervention versus health education control to reduce cognitive decline in older adults with hearing loss in the USA (ACHIEVE): a multicenter, randomized controlled trial. Lancet.

2023;402(10404):786-797. — ACHIEVE — landmark trial linking hearing intervention to cognitive protection.

2. Lin FR, Niparko JK, Ferrucci L. Hearing loss prevalence in the United States. Arch Intern Med. 2011;171(20):1851-1852. — U.S. hearing loss epidemiology.

3. Baguley D, McFerran D, Hall D. Tinnitus. Lancet. 2013;382(9904):1600-1607. — Authoritative tinnitus review.

Chapter 14 — The Gut: Your Digestive System

1. Katz PO, Dunbar KB, Schnoll-Sussman FH, Greer KB, Yadlapati R, Spechler SJ. ACG Clinical Guideline for the diagnosis and management of gastroesophageal reflux disease. Am J Gastroenterol. 2022;117(1):27-56. — ACG GERD guideline.

2. Rinninella E, Raoul P, Cintoni M, et al. What is the healthy gut microbiota composition? A changing ecosystem across age, environment, diet, and diseases. Microorganisms. 2019;7(1):14. — Comprehensive gut microbiome review.

3. Strate LL, Morris AM. Epidemiology, pathophysiology, and treatment of diverticulitis. Gastroenterology. 2019;156(5):1282-1298.e1. — Authoritative diverticulitis review.

4. Bharucha AE, Lacy BE. Mechanisms, evaluation, and management of chronic constipation. Gastroenterology. 2020;158(5):1232-1249.e3. — Authoritative constipation review.

5. Lacy BE, Pimentel M, Brenner DM, et al. ACG Clinical Guideline: management of irritable bowel syndrome. Am J Gastroenterol. 2021;116(1):17-44. — Current ACG IBS guideline.

6. US Preventive Services Task Force; Davidson KW, Barry MJ, Mangione CM, et al. Screening for colorectal cancer: US Preventive Services Task Force recommendation statement. JAMA. 2021;325(19):1965-1977. — Current USPSTF CRC screening recommendation (now starting at 45).

7. Valdes AM, Walter J, Segal E, Spector TD. Role of the gut microbiota in nutrition and health. BMJ. 2018;361:k2179. — Plain-language microbiome discussion.

Chapter 15 — Kidney and Urinary Tract Issues

1. Kidney Disease: Improving Global Outcomes (KDIGO) CKD Work Group. KDIGO 2024 Clinical Practice Guideline for the Evaluation and Management of Chronic Kidney Disease. Kidney Int. 2024;105(4S):S117-S314. — Current KDIGO CKD guideline; the authoritative CKD reference.

2. Heerspink HJL, Stefánsson BV, Correa- Rotter R, et al; DAPA-CKD Trial Committees and Investigators. Dapagliflozin in patients with chronic kidney disease. N Engl J Med. 2020;383(15):1436-1446. — DAPA-CKD — foundational SGLT2-CKD trial (includes non-diabetic patients).

3. The EMPA-KIDNEY Collaborative Group; Herrington WG, Staplin N, Wanner C, et al. Empagliflozin in patients with chronic kidney disease. N Engl J Med. 2023;388(2):117-127. — EMPA-KIDNEY — SGLT2 CKD trial across broader CKD population.

4. US Preventive Services Task Force; Grossman DC, Curry SJ, Owens DK, et al. Screening for prostate cancer: US Preventive Services Task Force recommendation statement. JAMA.

2018;319(18):1901-1913. — PSA screening recommendation; supports shared decision-making discussion.

5. Andriole GL, Crawford ED, Grubb RL 3rd, et al; PLCO Project Team. Prostate cancer screening in the randomized Prostate, Lung, Colorectal, and Ovarian Cancer Screening Trial: mortality results after 13 years of follow-up. J Natl Cancer Inst. 2012;104(2):125-132. — Foundational PSA screening trial.

6. Lerner LB, McVary KT, Barry MJ, et al. Management of lower urinary tract symptoms attributed to benign prostatic hyperplasia: AUA guideline part I — initial work-up and medical management. J Urol. 2021;206(4):806-817. — Current AUA BPH guideline.

7. Scales CD Jr, Smith AC, Hanley JM, Saigal CS; Urologic Diseases in America Project. Prevalence of kidney stones in the United States. Eur Urol. 2012;62(1):160-165. — U.S. kidney stone epidemiology.

Chapter 16 — The Immune System and Aging

1. Franceschi C, Garagnani P, Parini P, Giuliani C, Santoro A. Inflammaging: a new immune-metabolic viewpoint for age-related diseases. Nat Rev Endocrinol. 2018;14(10):576-590. — Review on inflammaging; current reference for the concept.

2. Goronzy JJ, Weyand CM. Understanding immunosenescence to improve responses to vaccines. Nat Immunol. 2013;14(5):428-436. — Supports immunosenescence and vaccine- response sections.

3. Cunningham AL, Lal H, Kovac M, et al; ZOE-70 Study Group. Efficacy of the herpes zoster subunit vaccine in adults 70

years of age or older. N Engl J Med. 2016;375(11):1019-1032. — Shingrix (zoster) efficacy trial in older adults.

4. Belkaid Y, Hand TW. Role of the microbiota in immunity and inflammation. Cell. 2014;157(1):121-141. — Supports microbiome-immune section.

Chapter 17 — Your Breathing Apparatus

1. Peppard PE, Young T, Barnet JH, Palta M, Hagen EW, Hla KM. Increased prevalence of sleep-disordered breathing in adults. Am J Epidemiol. 2013;177(9):1006-1014. — Foundational OSA prevalence data.

2. McEvoy RD, Antic NA, Heeley E, et al; SAVE Investigators and Coordinators. CPAP for prevention of cardiovascular events in obstructive sleep apnea. N Engl J Med. 2016;375(10):919-931. — Supports sleep-apnea section.

3. Chung F, Abdullah HR, Liao P. STOP- Bang Questionnaire: a practical approach to screen for obstructive sleep apnea. Chest. 2016;149(3):631-638. — Practical for patient screening.

4. US Preventive Services Task Force; Krist AH, Davidson KW, Mangione CM, et al. Interventions for tobacco smoking cessation in adults, including pregnant persons: US Preventive Services Task Force recommendation statement. JAMA. 2021;325(3):265-279. — USPSTF smoking-cessation intervention recommendation.

Chapter 18 — The Mind Matters: Navigating Mental Health in Aging

1. Holt-Lunstad J, Smith TB, Baker M, Harris T, Stephenson D. Loneliness and social isolation as risk factors for mortality: a meta-analytic review. Perspect Psychol Sci. 2015;10(2):227-237. — Foundational meta-analysis on loneliness and mortality.

2. Emmons RA, McCullough ME. Counting blessings versus burdens: an experimental investigation of gratitude and subjective well being in daily life. J Pers Soc Psychol. 2003;84(2):377-389. — Foundational gratitude-and-wellbeing study.

3. Kabat-Zinn J. Full Catastrophe Living: Using the Wisdom of Your Body and Mind to Face Stress, Pain, and Illness. Rev. ed. New York, NY: Bantam; 2013. — Foundational text on mindfulness-based stress reduction (MBSR).

4. Lee LO, James P, Zevon ES, et al. Optimism is associated with exceptional longevity in 2 epidemiologic cohorts of men and women. Proc Natl Acad Sci U S A. 2019;116(37):18357-18362. — Optimism-and-longevity study; supports the optimism section.

5. Conwell Y, Van Orden K, Caine ED. Suicide in older adults. Psychiatr Clin North Am. 2011;34(2):451-468. — Authoritative review on suicide in older adults.

Chapter 19 — Experimental Aging Remedies

1. López-Otín C, Blasco MA, Partridge L, Serrano M, Kroemer G. Hallmarks of aging: an expanding universe. Cell. 2023;186(2):243-278. — Updated "hallmarks of aging" framework — essential conceptual reference for this chapter.

2. Blackburn EH, Epel ES, Lin J. Human telomere biology: a contributory and interactive factor in aging, disease risks, and protection. Science. 2015;350(6265):1193-1198. — Authoritative Blackburn telomere review (Nobel laureate); supports telomere section.

3. Barzilai N, Crandall JP, Kritchevsky SB, Espeland MA. Metformin as a tool to target aging. Cell Metab. 2016;23(6):1060-1065. — TAME trial rationale paper from Nir Barzilai; supports metformin/longevity discussion.

4. Manson JE, Cook NR, Lee IM, et al; VITAL Research Group. Vitamin D supplements and prevention of cancer and cardiovascular disease. N Engl J Med. 2019;380(1):33-44. — Supports the vitamin-D-and-omega-3 section.

5. Bischoff-Ferrari HA, Vellas B, Rizzoli R, et al; DO-HEALTH Research Group. Effect of vitamin D supplementation, omega-3 fatty acids, and a strength- training exercise program on clinical outcomes in older adults: the DO- HEALTH randomized clinical trial. JAMA. 2020;324(18):1855-1868. — Supports the "omega-3/vitamin D/exercise" recommendation.

6. Laukkanen T, Khan H, Zaccardi F, Laukkanen JA. Association between sauna bathing and fatal cardiovascular and all-cause mortality events. JAMA Intern Med. 2015;175(4):542-548. — Landmark Finnish sauna-and-longevity study.

7. Kirkland JL, Tchkonia T. Senolytic drugs: from discovery to translation. J Intern Med. 2020;288(5):518-536. — Senolytics review from the Mayo group that pioneered the field.

8. Mattson MP, Longo VD, Harvie M. Impact of intermittent

fasting on health and disease processes. Ageing Res Rev. 2017;39:46-58. — Authoritative fasting- and-health review.

Chapter 20 — Artificial Intelligence (AI) and the Future of Medicine

1. Topol EJ. High-performance medicine: the convergence of human and artificial intelligence. Nat Med. 2019;25(1):44-56. — Topol's foundational frame-of- reference review for AI in medicine.

2. Rajpurkar P, Chen E, Banerjee O, Topol EJ. AI in health and medicine. Nat Med. 2022;28(1):31-38. — Updated AI-in-medicine review.

3. Esteva A, Kuprel B, Novoa RA, et al. Dermatologist-level classification of skin cancer with deep neural networks. Nature. 2017;542(7639):115-118. — Landmark AI-matches-dermatologist paper; cited in nearly all AI-medicine discussions.

4. McKinney SM, Sieniek M, Godbole V, et al. International evaluation of an AI system for breast cancer screening. Nature. 2020;577(7788):89-94. — Landmark AI mammography paper; supports early-cancer-detection claim.

5. World Health Organization. Ethics and Governance of Artificial Intelligence for Health: WHO Guidance. Geneva: WHO; 2021. — WHO guidance on AI in health; directly supports the health-equity and risks sections.

6. Obermeyer Z, Powers B, Vogeli C, Mullainathan S. Dissecting racial bias in an algorithm used to manage the health of populations. Science. 2019;366(6464):447-453. — Foundational paper on algorithmic racial bias in health care.

7. Adamson AS, Smith A. Machine learning and health care disparities in dermatology. JAMA Dermatol. 2018;154(11):1247-1248. — Cited for the "skin cancer algorithms fail on darker skin" example.

8. Singhal K, Azizi S, Tu T, et al. Large language models encode clinical knowledge. Nature. 2023;620(7972):172- 180. — Foundational LLM-in-medicine paper; supports the chatbots/AGI discussion.

www.ingramcontent.com/pod-product-compliance
Lightning Source LLC
LaVergne TN
LVHW010649110826
845149LV00014B/2999

* 9 7 9 8 9 9 6 0 1 6 2 0 4 *